ORGANIZATION AND MANAGEMENT
OF
HOSPITAL LABORATORIES

ORGANIZATION AND MANAGEMENT

OF

HOSPITAL LABORATORIES

A. P. JOHNSON

F.I.M.L.T., GRAD. MEM. I.P.M.

Chief Technician, Department of Pathology, West Wales General Hospital; Lecturer in Chemical Pathology, Pibwrlwyd Technical College, Carmarthen; Visiting Lecturer, Kings Fund, College of Hospital Management, London

LONDON

BUTTERWORTHS

ENGLAND:	BUTTERWORTH & CO. (PUBLISHERS) LTD. LONDON: 88 Kingsway, W.C.2
AUSTRALIA:	BUTTERWORTH & CO. (AUSTRALIA) LTD. SYDNEY: 20 Loftus Street MELBOURNE: 343 Little Collins Street BRISBANE: 240 Queen Street
CANADA:	BUTTERWORTH & CO. (CANADA) LTD. TORONTO: 14 Curity Avenue, 374
NEW ZEALAND:	BUTTERWORTH & CO. (NEW ZEALAND) LTD. WELLINGTON: 49/51 Ballance Street AUCKLAND: 35 High Street
SOUTH AFRICA:	BUTTERWORTH & CO. (SOUTH AFRICA) LTD. DURBAN: 33/35 Beach Grove

Suggested U.D.C. Number: 362.11.006.2
Suggested Additional Number: 616–09.006.2

Standard Book Number 407 34650 3

Made and printed in Great Britain
at the St Ann's Press, Park Road, Altrincham

CONTENTS

FOREWORD

The management of hospital laboratories is a complex subject and varies greatly from hospital to hospital.

As a hospital exists for the treatment of its patients, a hospital laboratory plays an essential role in this existence. Communication therefore is vital, and the laboratory must be able to communicate the results of its tests as quickly and efficiently as possible. The method by which this is achieved may suit one laboratory but may not be the best for another.

Different staffing structures can create problems in one Laboratory that are not in others.

Because of these and many more variables it is not an easy task to write a book on the Management of Hospital Laboratories without it becoming a catalogue of techniques for handling equipment, stores and orders.

In this book Mr. Johnson has not tried to lay down hard and fast rules, but has attempted, and I think succeeded in, an explanation of the relationships that must develop between managers, generally Chief Technicians, and other staff, and the background knowledge that managers must have, to enable them to run an efficient laboratory.

I personally feel that managers are born and not made, but I believe that all will benefit and become a little better after reading this book.

F. J. BAKER

PREFACE

The aim of this book is to examine the development of pathology departments and the staff who work in them in order to provide some guide line for people who have to run such departments. My interest in management arose when I was appointed chief technician to a group of highly individualistic pathology departments scattered in a rural area. It soon became clear that technical training alone was not enough here; although a study of the literature on management techniques produced a number of ideas that could usefully be applied in pathology departments, my early attempts at applying these was less successful than I had anticipated. At this stage, I was invited to join an experimental management course by John Phillips, Staff Officer to the Welsh Hospital Board. Miss A. Crichton, a member of the academic staff of the University of South Wales and Monmouthshire, who was the course tutor, aroused my interest in the social sciences and thus provided the missing piece in the 'jigsaw' of departmental management. It was when I came to use this new knowledge that I realized that an appreciation of the development of these departments and the professional groups was essential to an understanding of the current situation and to the successsful application of managerial skills.

My description and analysis of an average pathology department has inevitably been influenced by my personal experience just as has my knowledge of management been influenced by those who taught me this subject. A number of chief technicians and pathologists have been kind enough to invite me to visit their departments thus widening my experience. My activities in the Association of Scientific Workers and lecturing I have done on departmental management have helped me to take a balanced view both of 'labour' and of 'management'. However, the speed at which pathology and management are developing has made it difficult in writing to cover the total range of new trends in this sphere.

Initially I assumed the book would be of interest only to pathologists, biochemists and technicians but discussions with a number of people have convinced me that hospital secretaries, regional board planners and training officers and heads of other hospital departments may also find it useful.

It is a tradition, which I gladly follow, to acknowledge any help received. The greatest assistance was given to me by C. B. Fisher, chief technician at Bronglais Hospital, Aberystwyth who read all the drafts and made valuable criticisms and suggestions. D. Slade read the final draft and helped in correcting some of the detail. E. Long kindly provided documents and information about the early days of the Institute. Dr. D. F. Davies and other members of the staff in the pathology department, West Wales General Hospital discussed many of the ideas in the book with me, though this does not imply that they agree with all of them. The views expressed and any mistakes are entirely my own responsibility. The final draft was read by some members of the Kings Fund College of Hospital Management who offered several helpful suggestions. Mrs. J. Johnson patiently converted the original rambling draft into readable prose; Mrs. J. Tolman and Mrs. A. Jones, typed the final draft. I have to thank the South West Wales Hospital Management Committee for permission to publish the book. Finally the publishers have earned my thanks for their help in the presentation and final corrections.

A. P. JOHNSON

CHAPTER 1

THE FUNCTION AND STRUCTURE
OF PATHOLOGY DEPARTMENTS

INTRODUCTION

The term management means different things to different people. To any technician primarily concerned with scientific work it must inevitably suggest something vaguely unpleasant but unavoidable in the form of paper work and administration. Some of the older generation of technicians may see it as a conflict—a sort of demarcation dispute or competition for power between pathologist and chief technician—and, in result, are fearful of the consequences. To the pathologist whose main interest is in diagnostic work and consultancy, however, it means a tedious round of meetings, letters, staff problems and struggles for money. Although much of the time of pathologists and chief technicians is still taken up with medical and scientific work, which they enjoy and find satisfying, nevertheless a considerable part is occupied with the running of the department. This work is often regarded as being quite unrelated to scientific work and as having no clear pattern of activity or defined goal and therefore as something of a frustrating burden.

Some chief technicians and pathologists will question the need for a book on the management of pathology departments since they consider that they have been running them successfully for a long time and will continue to do so. Again, some will feel such a book unnecessary because they believe that the term management is synonymous with administration and paper work which is best learnt by experience. There are many, though, who are not satisfied with the way in which they are running their department nor are they happy about meeting future increases in work. There is a growing feeling that the management of pathology departments should be brought into sharper focus and examined in detail as the precise purpose of these departments is not always clear.

Because departmental management is still only in the descriptive phase of development, it is not possible to write a textbook on the subject. There are no theories of management that can be taught.

Medical technology must merge into managerial activities and there can be no clear division. While a technician may know how to estimate a blood urea in 3 different ways, he may not know the best way of estimating 30 blood ureas a day for 52 weeks a year or 50 on one day and 10 on the next. Similarly, a pathologist will be able to distinguish between an adenocarcinoma and an epithelioma but may experience difficulty in deciding whether to develop techniques concerned with auto-immune diseases or with exfoliative cytology when there is only enough money to finance development in one of these.

Clearly then, in many ways, management can be considered as an activity concerned with solving problems. Progress and change in pathology departments, as in every field of medicine and science, have been such that it is necessary to look at the whole picture to see how well problems are being solved. In any organization that is growing rapidly, deficiencies that were initially not obvious or important become so and tend to threaten future growth. Problems created by growth do not differ to any great extent whether they arise in pathology, the National Health Service (N.H.S.), the trade unions or in industry generally. Pathologists and technicians watching television programmes on management skills in industry will recognize, from their own experience, many of the situations used in such programmes.

The N.H.S. is some 21 years old and there seems now to be a temporary pause before the introduction of major changes, so this is a good time to look at the organization and management of pathology departments. Many will remember the major problems in 1947 in obtaining accurate results from estimations and they will appreciate the satisfactory progress that has been made in this —a technical problem capable of being solved by people trained in technology. Today the problems are different as they are concerned not with medical science or technology but rather with matters of organization, with recruiting people and with making the best use of skill and money which are both in short supply. They are, in consequence, not problems to be solved by people trained in medicine or technology but managerial problems which require different knowledge and skills. It is now a matter of urgency to include some form of management training in the general education of pathologists, biochemists and technicians. To find out what should be taught it is important to analyse the work done by these three groups in their respective jobs, to ascertain what the hospital expects of them and to identify the various skills

2

and knowledge required so as to build these into the course of studies of the three groups.

It is not only change within pathology departments that is important. When they came into being in general hospitals, they were strongly influenced by the design and function of similar departments in teaching hospitals, and tended to be used by clinicians in the same way. Today clinicians are using pathology departments differently and general practitioners are using them as well. All this makes it necessary for the top team of pathologists and chief technicians to reconsider the way in which their department is organized, staffed, financed and equipped.

The environment within the N.H.S. has altered considerably since 1947; the Ministry of Health* now exercises considerable direct influence, and Regional Boards are considering centralization and inter Hospital Group co-operation. In the immediate future major changes are envisaged within the N.H.S. in a number of reports by Farqueshon-Lang, Hunt, Salmon and Cogwheel (Reports 1966 a, b, c and 1967 respectively) and in 1968 the Ministry of Health published, for discussion, a green paper on the re-organization of the N.H.S. (Ministry of Health, 1968b). The Hospital Services Organization and Management Report No. 10 (Ministry of Health, 1967) has described the internal organization of pathology departments and refers to the chief technician as the departmental manager.

As any organism grows larger, its internal structure becomes more complex, specialized and highly organized so that it is necessary to expend more energy on maintaining its internal environment. If it is to survive and flourish, the organism must be capable of detecting changes in its external environment, correctly assessing their significance and producing the correct adaptive response or it will fail to thrive. The same is true of pathology departments for those who administer them must detect change in the needs of clinicians, the policy of the Ministry of Health, the Regional Board and the Hospital Management Committee and changes, too, in technology and, having accurately assessed the significance of such changes, produce the correct response or such departments will not thrive. More effort should go into the servicing of the internal environment of the department, having regard not only to equipment but also to people working in it and to the lines of communication which may become ineffective and prone to interference as the department grows larger. Sociological problems

---

*Now known as the Department of Health and Social Security (D.H.S.S.)

arise as numbers of staff increase, for informal but powerful groups appear who may not see things in the same way as the pathologist or chief technician. This again creates new activities for the top team and new problems requiring knowledge, understanding and skill outside the orbit of their professional training.

Without attempting to find a precise definition of management the majority would agree that here it implies a complex activity of organizing a pathology department to be (a) effective—that is, to achieve its purpose; and (b) efficient—that is, to make the best use of available human and material resources. To do this senior staff must have a clear idea of the purpose of their department and of how it is related to the hospital as a whole. The first two chapters, then, analyse the activities of an 'average' pathology department in a District General Hospital and establish a criteria of effectiveness. They also describe the development of the three professions and examine some of their current attitudes and aspirations. Chapters 4, 5 and 6 are concerned with managerial and social skills that are used in administering departments. The early chapters will interest hospital administrators and planners.

THE PURPOSE OF PATHOLOGY DEPARTMENTS

The purpose of pathology departments has been variously described as: 'the identification of the origins of ill health; the way in which extrinsic and intrinsic factors distort the physical and mental patterns of the normal persons are the business of the clinical pathologists . . . ' ; 'Clinical pathology may be defined as that field of medical activity covering the application through the instrumentality of the hospital laboratory, of its basic science to the clinical practise of medicine both in diagnosis and treatment of Disease' (*see* Leading Article in the *Journal of Clinical Pathology,* 1967); 'The purpose of clinical pathology is thus practical, its immediate aim is the care of the patient . . . ' ; 'Clinical pathology is the care and welfare of the patient' (Dyke, 1964). The pathology department is commonly described as providing a diagnostic service although evidence suggests that this is not an accurate picture of its function. Generally speaking, from the various definitions that have been written two points emerge as common, firstly, it is a diagnostic service and secondly it is for the benefit of the patient. Unfortunately this definition does not help laboratory staff when they try to assess how good is the service they are providing and if it is adequate, so it is necessary to analyse more closely just what a pathology department does and so ascertain its true purpose.

To start with the simplest possible description—a clinician sends in a request to the department with a specimen or with a patient and expects a report. Although the clinician may write the name of a test on the request form, he is really asking for information and is not usually concerned how the information is obtained or which technique is used to provide it and indeed in some instances laboratory staff may know a better test in a given condition.

Clinicians Who Use Pathology Departments

Clinicians using pathology departments fall into three groups, hospital clinicians, general practitioners and medical officers of health. Of the hospital clinicians, house officers probably initiate 70 per cent of the pathology requests, registrars about 25 per cent and consultants 5 per cent. It is therefore, worth considering some of the common characteristics of house officers since they use the department most frequently. Between 50 and 60 per cent of them are not British, and English is not their primary language; they have a different social background and different social values in consequence. A house officer stays in a post for 6 months only and it is unusual for him to receive a formal introduction to the various hospital departments (including the pathology department). It is uncommon, too, to find methods and procedures laid down regarding the way in which the ancillary services are to be used. In result a new house officer joining the hospital staff will not know the work programme of the pathology department nor will he have been given much guidance as to how to use the services of the pathology department. He is merely another strange voice on the telephone and by the time the laboratory staff get to know him it is almost time for him to change his job. All house officers will have been encouraged, as medical students, to learn by investigation and while facilities in medical schools are such as to be able to cope with the resulting flood of pathology requests this is not so in the average District General Hospital.

The general practitioners, on an average, provide 10 per cent of pathology requests—mainly for haematology, and requiring relatively simple answers, and it is unusual for them to ask for the more complicated tests that are available. A survey has indicated the variation in the requirements of general practitioners and some of the reasons for them (Darmady, 1964). It is probably fair to say that a percentage of pathology requests are concerned

5

with the continued training of housemen as it is now widely recognized that they are still in training.

The final group, who are responsible for approximately 5 per cent of pathology requests at present coming into pathology departments, are medical officers of health (M.O.H.). In 1947 when the N.H.S. was created, they lost the laboratories which they had under the Local Authorities. With the marked decrease in infectious diseases, their jobs became less clear. More recently an interest in preventive medicine, which lies in the field of the M.O.H., has been growing and they are now looking for methods of screening normal populations. For this the Medical Officer must have the services of pathology departments but the services are scarce and invariably located in hospitals. The demands of clinicians are given much higher priority. There have only been a few pilot schemes in recent years in which the M.O.H. has been given facilities in pathology departments for screening normal populations. Neither the general practitioner nor the M.O.H. has been made particularly welcome; access to laboratory facilities had to be facilitated by a directive from the Ministry of Health. Most pathologists feel, with justification, that they have their hands full with work coming in from hospitals and that there is not enough money or staff to go round.

Why Clinicians Use Pathology Departments

It is worth considering why clinicians ask for pathological investigation beside the genuine need for information and to follow the effects of treatment and screening. Probably the most common reason among housemen is to anticipate the questions which the consultant may possibly ask on his round later. Often it may be a matter of so-called routine or (even more open to criticism) that the clinician has read about a new test in a recent medical journal. Some housemen may have no clear idea of what they are looking for and hope that one of the tests will produce some useful information to aid in diagnosis. The housemen have at their command a powerful diagnostic and therapeutic organization which they are expected to call into action when they feel it necessary. Lack of diagnostic experience and uncertainty about his superior's reactions to his decisions encourages him to ask for the maximum amount of information about his patient's condition (for example, pathology reports) to compensate for any lack of confidence. A houseman more forthcoming than many—when asked about the value of a long list of pathology requests for a patient admitted late at night with acute abdominal pains—conceded that the reports would serve rather to prop up his sagging confidence than to benefit the patient.

How Clinicians Use Pathology Departments

Evidence suggests that pathology departments are overworked but that the best use is not being made of their facilities. Certainly pathologists feel that they are being swamped by the excessive use of their departments. Part of this failure to modify demands is inherent in the education of doctors, who are not taught to consider the financial consequences of their action, their outlook being bound up in the concept of clinical freedom. To give just two examples of this extravagant use of the service, Gould (1966) found that only one-quarter of patients were given antibiotic therapy depending on bacteriological advice and there appeared to be little difference in the results of the treatment whether this advice was used or not. Tests for antibiotic sensitivity were found to require 20 per cent of technical time in bacteriology laboratories. Again, at the present time over the country as a whole, approximately 14 per cent of all blood issued to hospital laboratories is returned unused—and usually out of date—to transfusion centres. It is probable that most of this blood has been cross-matched with a view to use during surgery. Thus a Leading Article in the *British Medical Journal* of 1957 points out: 'often blood is requested solely because the house-man is not clear about his chief's requirements and so cross-matches an excess to make sure'. Some clinicians recognize this state of affairs for Cook (1967) comments:

> Consultants must accept their fair share of blame in the abuse of these ancillary investigations. With so many laboratory facilities and all manner of superb radiological aids to hand, they too readily resort to these and more elaborate methods before they have tried to get as near to the truth as possible without them . . . I would add, tormented the patient by innumerable tiresome and often unnecessary investigations which can be painful, even frankly dangerous, quite apart from the cost to the service in man power and bed usage with the inevitable delay imposed on others.

Clinicians send routine work to pathology departments between the hours of 9 a.m. and 5 p.m., apart from minor local variations. There are two other ways in which pathology departments undertake work. The first is that of pathologists attending the patients in

7

their own homes at the request of a general practitioner, collecting a blood sample and bringing this back to the department where the work is done as part of the department routine. Not every one of these domiciliary visits seems to involve a consultation or advice.

The second further facility is the emergency service available after 5 p.m., or whenever the department closes, until 9 a.m. the next morning. This originated in blood-transfusion laboratories but the system spread to pathology departments early in 1950, in the form of an 'on-call' service. Payment is made to technicians being called out. With changes in medical practice clinicians, particularly house officers, have come to rely on pathology reports before taking any action; more blood is transfused and there is more concern about litigation by patients and this has all led to a greater use of the 'on-call' service. By 1964 the majority of pathology departments were actually operating a 24-hour service under the guise of an emergency 'on-call' service.

Looking back, then, over the past 21 years, it appears that the various laboratories in pathology departments have developed in response to the needs of clinicians and more recently to new advances in technology and equipment. In 1945 the bacteriology laboratory, the largest of the four laboratories, was the centre of the department. With the advent of antibiotics, the problems of treating infectious diseases diminished and its importance gradually declined. Then in the late 1940s the haematology laboratory became the centre and the most popular. Discoveries such as vitamin B_{12} and improved methods of classifying and identifying anaemias helped in its development. The first discussions of quality control were concerned with the commonest of all haematological investigations, the estimation of haemoglobin. This phase did not last long for by the mid-1950s biochemistry was taking first place as many exciting discoveries were made in this field and methods and equipment improved rapidly. Knowledge and skill rapidly accumulated in biochemistry laboratories and they have never looked back since. Some people have argued that in future all other laboratories will become subdivisions of biochemistry but this is unlikely in view of recent developments in immunology and cytogenetics.

There does not seem to have been any conscious planning in the development of pathology departments and there are still not many signs of this in 1969 apart from the call for more money and staff. The rate of change in technology is increasing and techniques which a few years ago would have been effected only by the chief technician are now rapidly passed down to junior staff. This transfer of skill now takes place faster than ever before and is due to better equipment, improved methods and certainly to pressure of work as well as to a change in attitude on the part of chief technicians. To a great extent the preparatory work, such as the preparation of reagents and equipment, is no longer carried out by students and greater use is being made of pre-packaged and disposable items. Pharmaceutical and chemical firms are offering kits of reagents for the latest techniques which makes it simpler to introduce them into routine use. Much of the repetitive work is now done by automatic equipment.

Many of the senior staff in charge of laboratories are keen to develop the scope of their own laboratories and are always prepared to try out new ideas in an effort to improve the service but at the same time to increase the size of their laboratory in relation to the others. Pathologists, on the other hand, are not entirely happy with the vast number of requests now reaching their departments. They are more interested in pathological problems in medical rather than in technical terms.

THE SUPPLY OF RESOURCES

Currently Regional Hospital Boards use a method of forecasting annual non-recurring expenditure for three years ahead. To this end pathology departments have had to submit forward-estimates for three years ahead for all items of non-recurring expenditure. Forward-estimates are collected from each hospital and passed to the group treasurer who collates them into a group forward-estimate for consideration by the Regional Board who then allocate money to the group—frequently less than the amount asked for. The reverse process then takes place, the group secretary allocates money to each hospital and the hospital secretary in turn allocates money to the various hospital departments. The system has not been satisfactorily explained to personnel and in some cases has even been tactfully ignored as some treasurers appear more interested in balancing their books than in using money as a positive form of management. As a result it rarely works as smoothly as this in practice, there is a lot of manoeuvering and in this case there appears to be some truth in the old adage 'he who shouts the loudest gets the most'. The money allocated in one year must be spent before the end of the financial year; otherwise it must be handed back to the Regional Board. There is a growing tendency for money for major equipment to be provided direct from Regional Boards. This is an interesting development and it is possible to foresee the grouping of a pathology service on a larger basis than that of a single H.M.C. to meet the growing needs of the G.P. and M.O.H. who do not provide money for the service at present.

In providing the money to meet the running costs of their pathology department, one of the checks on efficiency the H.M.C. uses is the unit cost and this gives some idea of how well the resources are being used; they also use the staff request ratio which gives an indication of how well staff is being used. This unit-cost system has been a bone of contention for many years and will continue to be so. Objection will continue to be raised to this and to Organization and Method studies, for like any other sort of worker, laboratory staff are reluctant to accept any investigation which might show that they are working less hard than they should be or that they are in any way responsible for inefficiency. The unit system is interpreted in widely different ways, the difficulty being the precise definition of a request and staff also find fault with the system for doing something badly that they feel it was never intended to do—that is, make an interdepartmental comparison of costs.

The hospital secretary is responsible for organizing a number of services for pathology departments—engineering, building maintenance, portering, cleaning and laundry. The hospital engineer and his staff maintain both services such as electricity, gas, water and heat and also equipment though the more complex equipment is often serviced under contract by manufacturers. The building supervisor and his staff are responsible for the fabric of the building, furniture and fittings. An assistant matron or domestic supervisor is responsible for the domestic staff cleaning the hospital. The hospital secretary—acting on behalf of the group secretary, chief executive officer of the employing authority (the H.M.C.)—recruits most grades of staff.

Pathology departments can obtain supplies and equipment through the central stores of the Ministry of Health, from manufacturers or suppliers on central or regional contracts or directly. In theory, small items costing less than twenty shillings and consumable items are ordered directly by chief technicians on local-purchase order forms though in practice this restriction is often ignored. Indents for larger items such as equipment are submitted via the hospital secretary or Group Medical Staff Committee to the group supplies officer who, in turn, submits them to the group finance committee for approval, after obtaining competitive quotations.

ORGANIZATION OF PATHOLOGY WITHIN THE N.H.S.

In theory, hospital secretaries transmit to pathology departments policy decisions and regulations from the H.M.C., from their Regional Board and from the Ministry of Health. In practice this line of communication is relatively ineffective for few departments ever see relevant Whitley Council circulars or Hospital Memorandum (H.M.) circulars issued by the Ministry. When the Ministry are planning policy for pathology departments they are advised by the Central Pathology Advisory Committee (C.P.A.C.) which is made up of pathologists from Regional Pathology Advisory Committees (R.P.A.C.). The Regional Committees have a co-ordinating function but do not appear to be very active. Advice offered by the C.P.A.C. is of interest to all senior laboratory staff working in pathology departments but the proceedings of the committee are not published and its minutes have a very restricted circulation. Resentment has been expressed by biochemists because they have no say in the formulation of policy for their laboratories at regional and national level.

There is no comparable line of communication for technicians though a Laboratory Technicians Consultative Committee was set up in 1958 to consider technical matters concerning the supply and quality of apparatus and equipment for use in hospital laboratories, and other relevant matters, and to make recommendations. Regional committees have been formed but with broader terms of reference and they discuss a wide range of matters of interest and concern to chief technicians.

Direction from the Ministry of Health is becoming surprisingly common. Some years ago there was a directive to H.M.C.'s to ensure that, as originally intended, general practitioners should have unlimited access to pathology departments. More recently the Ministry have laid down the amount of work a technician should be able to do in a year in terms of cytology slides, the first example of this occurring in 1967. They recommended that pathology departments should accept pregnancy tests from general practitioners suggesting not only the reagents but also the amount of a technician's time which would probably be spent doing this work. Again, the Ministry, after consulting the C.P.A.C., published Building and Equipment Notes for pathology departments setting out standards for size of departments and quantity of equipment. Unwilling as many pathologists are to accept central control, these Building and Equipment Notes have been accepted with enthu-

11

siasm because they ensure that the H.M.C. provides facilities at the recommended level. In the background there may be arguments about the accuracy of the notes or the level of the recommendations but they are used with conviction, if not always successfully.

SUPPLY OF SCIENTIFIC INFORMATION

As the primary function of the pathology department is to provide information for clinicians using technology, the staff must keep pace with the continual advances in medical science and the ever-changing technology. All departments receive or should receive a constant supply of up-to-date information in a form which is easily assimilated. An abundance of information is published in a great many journals and it is virtually impossible for staff to read them all in detail. Inevitably this means that occasionally new methods and techniques go unnoticed and often, in consequence, improved methods are introduced at too slow a rate. The main sources of information are books and journals and pathology departments can only afford a limited range of these. Reprints of articles are available but many technicians and pathologists have to pay for them. There is no circulation of information and no central library as there is in the Public Health Laboratory Service. The Hospital Centre organizes a packaged library service providing information taken from scientific journals covering non-technical matters of interest to pathology departments but these are relatively unknown. The Association of Clinical Patho-

TABLE 1

Staff Utilization

	Total annual requests in millions	Increase in requests each year expressed in millions	Increase in requests as a percentage of previous year	Request/technician ratio
1958	16	—	—	3,360
1959	17·2	1·2	7·5	3,500
1960	18·98	1·78	10·5	3,560
1961	20·6	1·62	8·5	3,720
1962	22·59	1·95	8·5	3,810
1963	24·93	2·4	10·5	4,000
1964	27·63	2·7	11	4,240
1965	28·56	0·93	3·5	4,070
1966	31·14	2·58	9	4,070

(Figures taken from Annual Reports of the Chief Medical Officer of the Ministry of Health (1958–1966) by courtesy of H.M.S.O.)

logists publish broadsheets on new techniques which have become accepted as good practice. The Association of Clinical Biochemists has published a number of circulars on equipment although these tend to be lists of equipment rather than reports of tests on each item. But all this is as yet inadequate and it is common enough to go into laboratories and find them using antiquated equipment and methods.

Information regarding scientific standards and official definitions are provided by national committees—as, for example, the nomenclature of the Rhesus blood-group system. Later definitions and standards are discussed and agreed at international level as in the case of haemoglobin standards, abnormal haemoglobin, the coagulation system and the classification of human chromosomes. Not all of these have been successfully agreed at international level, however, and some confusion has been caused concerning international units for enzymes, the Rhesus blood-group system and species and genera of micro-organisms.

HOW PATHOLOGY DEPARTMENTS USE RESOURCES

Turning for a moment to performance in pathology departments in terms of national figures, it has been almost impossible to make comparisons here and so detect trends, as the methods of recording performance have altered. The figures presented on unit cost for 1966–67 are in a form which is an improvement for heads of departments but less satisfactory for estimating national trends.

Since 1956 the annual number of requests has been rising steadily by some 10 per cent a year (*see* Table 1) and there is no evidence of an explosive increase even though total requests are a relatively crude indicator. It is difficult to decide whether this annual increase reflects a real increase in demand or simply an increase in capacity indicating an increasing investment in pathology services. It could also be an example of capacity increasing faster than demand and of the operation of one of Parkinson's Laws—that the work fills the time or capacity allotted to it. The number of requests per technician per annum have risen from 3,360 in 1958 to 4,070 in 1966 whilst at the same time the working week has decreased from 39 to 38 hours, holidays have increased, and day-release has been introduced. The average pathologist supervised 22,000 requests in 1958 and 30,000 in 1966. The total cost of pathology departments in England and Wales was approximately £15,000,000 in 1966 taking the average cost per 100 requests as £50. The breakdown of costs is shown in Table 2.

13

TABLE 2

Use of Resources in Pathology Departments
(Breakdown of Costs, 1964)

	Percentage of direct expenditure	Total cost in millions
Medical salaries	28	£3
Professional and technical salaries	47	£4·8
Domestic salaries	3·5	£0·4
Other salaries	2	£0·2
Drugs and dressings	1	£0·1
Equipment and supplies	15	£1·5
Other direct expenditure	3·5	£0·4

THE STAFF

Pathologists

Pathology departments are under the direction of consultant pathologists who constitute the second largest group (11 per cent of all consultants) in the N.H.S.; the total number has risen from 700 in 1956 to 939 in 1965—an average annual increase of 24. The normal method of recruitment is to place an advertisement in one of the professional journals. There is sometimes a link between a given pathology department and a pathology department in a particular teaching hospital but the greater the distance from the teaching hospitals the less likely the latter are to be interested in the appointment.

The House Officer receives an informal training while working in a pathology department as there is no specified syllabus. He continues to move up the ladder of appointments through Senior House Officer to Registrar, proceeding with his training, sometimes under the close supervision of a consultant pathologist and sometimes under the helpful guidance of a senior technician. The trainee pathologist will remain as a Registrar until he can find a post as a consultant. Until recently there were no appropriate higher qualifications for pathology, the Diploma in Pathology not being popular; in consequence some doctors acquired Membership of the Royal College of Physicians though it was not really suitable for their purpose; a larger number took an M.D.

The system described has many deficiencies and the post-qualification training has only recently been laid down by the College of Pathology although the examination for Membership of the

College had been running for some years. There have been complaints of training posts in pathology being used solely to recruit pairs of hands and so help to get the work done. The training and examination of the College seems to be directed at meeting a situation that existed ten years ago (though it hardly exists today), when pathologists were expected to be experts in technology. The present course of lectures for the I.M.L.T. Special Examination in Haematology would be suitable for anyone sitting for the Membership Examination of the College of Pathology. The emphasis on post-qualification training to obtain a higher qualification has led pathologists to tend to neglect the training in the skills they use daily in directing their department and upon which the success or quality of it is dependent.

Consultant pathologists are employed by the Regional Boards and are under the direction of the Senior Administrative Medical Officer. Contracts can be either full or part-time, allowance for private work being made in the latter case. Contracts in some regions do not specify how much time is to be spent respectively on N.H.S. work and on private work (Stevens, 1966). Pathologists are allowed to undertake private technical work in their department—one-third of the fee being taken by the H.M.C. and the other two-thirds being retained by the pathologist.

Career prospects in this field seem to be good at present as there are a sufficient number of pathologists in training (335 Registrars in 1965), to meet future vacancies and to maintain the present rate of growth of 27 extra consultant posts per year. Once appointed the pathologist has reached the top of the tree and there is no higher grading in spite of posts being designated both group and senior pathologist.

Biochemists

Biochemistry laboratories are often under the control of a biochemist who is either a science graduate or, less commonly, a pathologist. Entering the service with a first class honours degree a biochemist would be expected to serve at least two years in the probationary grade and another two years in the basic grade, both of which are considered as training posts. After this period he would be eligible for a senior grade. Advancement to Principal Biochemist depends on the size of the laboratory or on an outstanding performance and normally requires the approval of the Regional Board or even of the Ministry of Health.

In 1965 there were some 30 chemical pathologists and 330 biochemists (*see* Table 3). The breakdown shows 8 top grade, 40 principal and the rest senior basic and probationary grade biochemists.

TABLE 3

Numbers of Biochemists in Relation to Requests

Year	Biochemists	Requests per annum in millions
1957	204	
1958	197	16
1959	210	17·2
1960	228	18·98
1961	249	20·6
1962	265	22.59
1963	287	24·93
1964	299	27·63
1965	330	28.56

The figures must be judged against the 330 H.M.C. in England and Wales administering some 800 hospitals large enough to have pathology departments; this means that many biochemists in training posts are unsupervised. Biochemists are recruited straight from university or from within the service and most commonly by means of an advertisement in a scientific journal or the national press.

Prior to 1967 there was no particular post-qualification training for biochemists and a few took Ph.D. or M.Sc. but research degrees are not really suitable for biochemists in pathology departments where the accent is on providing a service for clinicians rather than on research. The Association of Clinical Biochemists, in conjunction with other bodies, has now established a Mastership in Clinical Biochemistry. Conditions of service are drawn up by a committee of the Whitley Council consisting of representatives of the management side and the staff side which includes the Association of Clinical Biochemists as well as trade unions.

Biochemists are employed by the relevant H.M.C. and have a normal contract but hours of work per week are not specified. Their rates of pay have been linked with those of university lecturers. Career prospects are good though the chance of reaching the top grade is small. A new entrant commences at £963 per annum and can expect to rise to £2,276 at the top of the senior grade with a maximum of 22 increments. This should be contrasted with the qualified technician who commences at £890 per annum and can rise to £2,175 with a maximum of 37 increments.

Technicians

Technicians are employed to carry on technological work in pathology departments. A new entrant, who must have four O-level passes, commences as a student technician and is upgraded to a junior after passing the Intermediate examination of the I.M.L.T. or the Ordinary National Certificate in Medical Laboratory Sciences. Promotion to technician grade depends on registration with the Medical Laboratory Technician Board, part of the Profession's Supplementary to Medicine Board. Junior technicians are eligible for registration on passing a final examination of the I.M.L.T. or a Higher National Certificate in Medical Laboratory Sciences or other specified subjects. Upgrading to senior 1 depends mainly on extra responsibility undertaken and on having passed two final I.M.L.T. examinations; and senior II on being in charge of 5 technical staff. Promotion to grades above senior I depends either on special responsibility or, more commonly, on the number of staff controlled. Thus a senior technician supervises a minimum of 5 technical staff, a chief I a staff of 8 or 11 if organized in separate departments and a chief II 20 or more.

In 1965 there were 7,020 technicians employed in the National Health Service, of whom 2,860 were qualified. The total number of technicians has been increasing by an average of 330 per year over the ten years until 1965 but in 1966 it increased by some 600 (*see* Table 4). No figures are available for the N.H.S. but analysis of the membership returns of the Institute show that an equal number of males and females have been recruited for the last ten years. In 1956 only 2 out of 10 women who passed the Intermediate examination also passed their first final examination. Ten years later this figure has risen to 5 women passing a first final out of every 10 taking the intermediate examination. Of women passing their first final in 1956 11 per cent were married and in 1966 21 per cent (*see* Table 5).

Regulations concerning training are laid down by the Institute of Medical Laboratory Technology who set the final and Intermediate examinations. The Joint Education Committee with members of the Department of Education and Science and the Institute set the syllabus and examination for the National Certificate courses. Standards of training and qualifications are set by the Medical Laboratory Technicians Board, part of the Profession's Supplementary to Medicine Council who define qualifications acceptable for the registration with the Board which is now a condition of service for technicians in the N.H.S. The Board also

17

TABLE 4
Technicians Employed in the N.H.S.
(1956–1966)

Year	Total	Qualified	Unqualified	Ratio of qualified to unqualified technicians
1956	4,349	2,281	2,068	1:0·9
1957	4,463	2,394	2,169	1:0·9
1958	4,758	2,439	2,317	1:0·95
1959	4,928	2,468	2,460	1:1
1960	5,316	2,729	2,587	1:0·95
1961	5,539	2,789	2,750	1:0·95
1962	5,939	2,985	2,949	1:1
1963	6,199	2,599	3,600	1:1·4
1964	6,516	2,702	3,814	1:1·4
1965	7,017	2,860	4,151	1:1·4
1966	7,631	3,097	4,534	1:1·5

TABLE 5
Ratio of Men to Women passing I.M.L.T. Examinations

	Total	Men (percentage)	Women (percentage)	Married women (percentage)
Intermediate examination				
1956	187	44	56	5
1966	392	42	58	6
Final examination for Associateship				
1956	526	70	30	11
1966	889	58	42	21

approves both new courses and pathology departments as suitable training establishments.

Students are recruited mainly from grammar schools with a minimum of four O-level passes but with a small percentage having one or more A-level passes. In many industrial areas recruitment is difficult because of competition from employers and the poor image that 'technicians' of any sort have in grammar schools. Youth employment officers, who are better informed than careers masters, do not seem to be much help in recruiting students. A few chief technicians attend careers conventions but results are not encouraging. The most widely used method of recruiting is to advertise in the local and national press or the I.M.L.T. Gazette though the average fifth former has no idea at all what a student technician is or what the Whitley Regulations imply. Qualified staff are recruited usually through the I.M.L.T. Gazette, by means of a stereotyped advertisement rarely giving at the time or offering on application a description of the job. The shortage of qualified technicians in the N.H.S. is often talked about and used as an excuse although there is not such a shortage in the country as a whole. In the last few years 600 juniors have passed their first final examination each year and become qualified technicians but the total number in the N.H.S. has increased only by 200 per annum, the rest being employed by industry, the Medical Research Council or Universities or—having married—women who leave to have children (*see* Table 6).

TABLE 6

	Increase in unqualified technicians in N.H.S.	*Total new students registered with I.M.L.T.*	*Increase in qualified technicians in N.H.S.*	*No. of new Associates in I.M.L.T.*
1957	101	641	113	—
1958	148	641	45	357
1959	153	842	29	338
1960	127	1,065	61	370
1961	163	1,036	60	360
1962	199	1,403	−4	400
1963	651	1,235	−386	532
1964	214	1,246	103	536
1965	343	1,857	158	687
1966	377	1,218	237	633

Students attend evening, day or block-release courses at technical college for a two- or three-year course leading to the Intermediate Examination of the I.M.L.T. or the Ordinary National Certificate Examination. A further two-year evening or day-release course leads either to a final examination of the I.M.L.T. or a Higher National Certificate in Medical Laboratory Sciences. Students usually spend six months in each of the four main laboratories gaining experience in technology before the Intermediate examination and then spend most of their time in one laboratory gaining experience in the chosen subject of their final examination.

Student technicians are employed on the understanding that they will receive training and experience which will enable them to sit the I.M.L.T. examination or National Certificates. School leavers are not unwilling to train but are put off to some extent by the low salaries offered in comparison with those received by their con-

19

temporaries. However, the main difficulty is that many pathology departments are unwilling to take training seriously and refuse to release students to attend lectures because of the pressure of work. Such departments have only sufficient staff to cope with the work-load and have rejected their training commitment. Small departments tend to train inefficiently and to have a high turnover of staff. Many pathology departments are even more unwilling to allow their staff to embark on National Certificate courses for this means students will attend technical college for 14 per cent of their annual work time on a day-release course and 18 per cent on a block-release course.

Before the introduction of National Certificate courses technicians had to pass the final examination of the Institute with a syllabus mainly based on techniques, the course lasting five years, though it was widely felt that this was too long. In any case the bulk of routine work in pathology departments is carried out by junior technicians—that is, those who have passed the Intermediate Examination. Few departments keep staff for long in the technicians grade as in such an event another department would soon offer him a higher grade to attract him. The five-year training has the disadvantage that the late starter would be in his mid or late twenties before earning a reasonable salary.

Career prospects for technicians are good and though the career grade is considered to be a senior II, most technicians assume they will reach chief I grade. There is a good deal of over-grading at present simply to retain skilled staff. It is usually easier to over-grade a technician than to increase the establishment. The starting salary of a chief technician has more than quadrupled between 1947 and 1967, from £420 to £1,700 per annum compared with a consultant pathologist's starting salary which has not even doubled over the same period, having risen from £1,700 to £3,200 per annum. The top of the scale for a chief technician II has increased at a slower rate than has that for other grades—98 per cent in ten years compared with 110 per cent for chief I and 116 per cent for senior II. This is probably because the top of the chief technician II scale is approaching that of senior administrative officers at group level—for example, deputy group secretaries.

Technicians' salaries and conditions of service are laid down nationally by the subcommittee of the Whitley Council consisting of representatives of the Ministry of Health, employing authorities and, representing technicians, trade unions. The organization and function of the Whitley Council will be considered in detail in the next chapter. Current conditions of service are described in the Whitley P.T.B. 'A' circular number 243.

INTERNAL ORGANIZATION OF PATHOLOGY DEPARTMENTS

It is now necessary to turn to a consideration of the internal organization of pathology departments. Each one is made up of four laboratories undertaking different types of work—bacteriology, biochemistry, haematology and histopathology. For the sake of clarity the term department will be used throughout to mean the four laboratories together and the term laboratory will be used to mean one section—for example, bacteriology.

Request forms and specimens are delivered from hospital wards, out-patient departments, general practitioners surgeries, and various local authority clinics to the reception which is usually part of the office in the pathology department. In some cases a patient will bring a request form directly and a member of the staff will collect a specimen from them. Clerical staff check the identity of the request form and specimen or patient as the case may be. They either record receipt in a register or, more commonly, record the test to be done and details of origin of the test material for the monthly record of work that has to be submitted to the records officer. The request and specimens are then sent to the appropriate laboratory.

Bacteriology

The bacteriology laboratory has the job of isolating and identifying micro-organisms and determining their sensitivity to a range of antibiotics. It also undertakes serological work to investigate the patients response to bacteriological infections. More recently the bacteriology laboratory has become involved in the investigation of cross-infection in hospitals and such things as checking the efficiency of autoclaving. Where the hospital has a central sterile supply department, the bacteriology laboratory may run their sterility control system. A few such laboratories in District General Hospitals will undertake virological work though this is not common. Staff are not able to predict work-loads and this can vary by plus or minus 50 per cent from day to day. Specimens arrive throughout the day but mainly between 9 a.m. and 10 a.m. and between 2 p.m. and 3 p.m. The range of tests is relatively small consisting mainly of swabs, urine, sputum and faeces for bacteriological culture and testing for antibiotic sensitivity. Techniques are

21

moving away from the elementary ones used for so long. Most of the culture media is now bought in dehydrated form rather than being made in the laboratory from basic ingredients as before. This is partly because dehydrated media is more consistent and partly because of pressure of work. There is little factual information about the comparative costs of the two media.

The general system is that specimens are cultured in the early afternoon and the culture read the following morning, the primary reports being sent out about midday. A small number of cultures will require further tests which may take from a few days to several weeks to complete, as for example, in the case of culture for tubercle bacilli. It appears that quality control of bacteriological methods is not common and little attempt is made to assess the efficiency of cultural methods for screening large numbers of specimens for a particular organism.

Haematology

The haematology laboratory undertakes, as the main part of its work, the counting of the cellular constituents of blood, the estimating of haemoglobin and the testing of the coagulation mechanisms of blood, together with a small number of specialized tests. The daily work-load varies by more than plus or minus 50 per cent and is increasing steadily by about 10–15 per cent per year. In some ways the work-load can be predicted as it is closely related to the activities of the clinical staff—for example, in the pre-operative round and antenatal clinics. Large laboratories use a flow system for the work, such as an autoanalyser, but more commonly the work is done in batches using mechanized equipment, electronic counters and machines for staining blood films. Quality control is well understood and widely used.

Blood Bank

The blood bank provides blood for transfusion to patients. It also undertakes blood grouping on surgical patients and on antenatal patients. The blood bank holds and controls the stocks of dried plasma, frozen plasma and fibrinogen. In fact, it acts as a sort of middleman between the Regional Blood Transfusion Units who supply these substances and the clinicians. Blood grouping is done by hand at present but attempts are being made to mechanize or automate this work. The standards for quality control have been largely set by the regional blood transfusion laboratories. Twenty years ago the standard of cross-matching blood was less than satisfactory and the regional laboratories insisted on very high standards with a view to improving the techniques used in hospital blood banks. Over the course of time the level of expertise in these banks has increased and because of the close contact with the clinician and patients, personnel have a better understanding of the implications of cross-matching techniques, the time taken and the needs of clinicians and patients. Regional Blood Transfusion centres, on the other hand, have remained isolated from clinicians and patients and still rigidly insist on rigorous standards in techniques for cross-matching. This is an interesting example of a centralized service continued to set standards though expertise and experience have become decentralized. A comparison between recommended methods of cross-matching in this country and those widely used on the continent give the impression that cross-matching is over-controlled in this country. The situation has been improved with the publication of a recommended method by the Association of Clinical Pathologists.

Chemical Pathology

The biochemistry laboratory carries out tests to provide information on the physiological mechanism of the body; the digestive system; homeostasis, organ functions and also the endocrine system. The information so obtained, as in the case of other laboratories, may be used to assist in diagnosis and to follow the effects of treatment, medical or surgical. The daily work-load varies by plus or minus 50 per cent and is increasing by about 10 per cent per annum. The average biochemistry laboratory offers a range of 30–40 tests but approximately 90 per cent of the requests coming in involve the use of small groups of 9–11 tests. The range of tests is very dependent on the scientific interests of the staff in the laboratory. Quality control is widely used but in spite of this, precision and accuracy vary widely from one biochemistry laboratory to another as recent surveys show. Twenty years ago there was probably some inefficiency shown up by quality control but today quality control is showing up laboratories who, because of pressure of work, have chosen a method of screening samples to distinguish between low, normal or high results rather than accurately estimating a substance. More recently two other methods of control have been introduced—cumulative summation and distribution curves of results of estimations—which give a better picture of the total accuracy of the techniques and of the staff carrying out the estimations.

23

Histology

The histology laboratory prepares sections of tissue to be examined by a pathologist. In the last few years they have been undertaking screening of cytology smears for the detection of malignant cells. This work is mainly carried out by technicians who look at the slides and write and sign the reports on the smears.

The Office

Once a request has been completed the written report is sent to the department's office where it is processed by the clerical staff. This processing may involve separating N.C.R. duplicate forms, typing a copy from the written report or photocopying it. The top copy is dispatched to the clinician who sent in the request and the duplicate copies are filed. Some departments retrieve previous reports and attach them to another request for the same patient though this practice is declining. In 1967 a small number of pathology departments stopped filing copies of reports other than histology reports, but other laboratories began investigating the advantages of mechanical handling and analysis of reports. The system of checking reports varies; a few years ago the majority of pathology departments had the same system in which reports were saved until the late afternoon when the pathologist checked and signed them before they were dispatched. This system is beginning to change for a variety of reasons, mainly because of pressure of work and in some departments senior technicians and biochemists in charge of laboratories are signing reports before they go to the office. As many as 95 per cent of reports leaving some departments will not have been seen by a pathologist. In 1959, 780 pathologists supervised 17 million requests—just over 20,000 requests per pathologist per year. In 1965 each pathologist supervised approximately 30,000 per year.

The clerical staff are usually women and the senior acts as a private secretary to the senior pathologist; she consequently wields considerable power and in many ways has better communications and more influence with the pathologist than has his chief technician.

SUMMARY

This chapter has attempted a brief description of pathology departments—discussing their purpose, their relationship with the hospital, their internal organization and the people who work in them. It illustrates that a pathology department is not simply an organization into which a clinician pushes a request and gets out the answer (Thus the diagram here (*Figure 1*) represents an oversimplification).

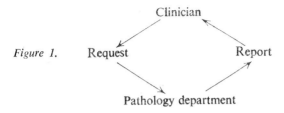

Figure 1.

Figure caption / labels: Clinician, Request, Report, Pathology department

For there are a number of other essential activities that have to be undertaken to achieve even this limited purpose, such as obtaining resources from the H.M.C. (and feeding back information about performance to them), and recruiting and training staff. The major purpose and the secondary activities are achieved

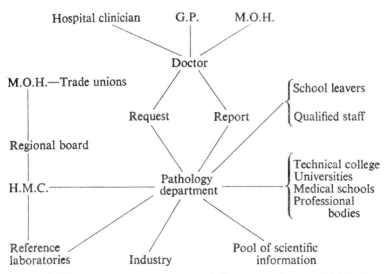

Figure 2. Diagrammatic representation of the personnel and official bodies involved in the functioning of a pathology department.

within constraints imposed by the Ministry of Health, Regional Boards, H.M.C., professional bodies, other hospital departments competing for money and other employers competing for qualified staff (*see Figure 2*).

CHAPTER 2

DEVELOPMENT OF PATHOLOGISTS, TECHNICIANS AND BIOCHEMISTS

INTRODUCTION

The purpose of this chapter is to outline the development of pathology, of hospital organization and of the three groups of professional personnel involved and to demonstrate the interplay between medical practice, technology and the professional aspirations of these three groups. This is not an attempt to provide a detailed history but only to highlight the salient points. Most of the information was derived from journals and annual reports of the Association of Clinical Pathologists, The College of Pathology, The Association of Clinical Biochemists and the Institute of Medical Laboratory Technology as well as medical journals.

Staff and in turn pathology departments are influenced by the way in which clinicians use the department and also by changes in the environment within hospitals and the N.H.S. and in government policy. Staff have to adopt strategies which will enable them to survive and flourish and either to counteract or adapt to changes in the needs of the clinician or in environment. Therefore—in order to understand the present position in pathology departments and the attitudes and behaviour of the staff—it is useful to look at the origins of the latter, and the forces that have influenced their development. Causes can then be sought for seemingly irrational behaviour instead of dismissing it. The reasons for technicians resisting shift work and pathologists feeling their work cannot be measured, may not be obvious but perhaps some clues can be found while surveying their development as professional groups. It may be equally rewarding to look at the influences that have shaped the structure of pathology departments as this might throw some light on the question of the appropriateness of the present organizational structure to the task as it is today.

The person in charge of a pathology department has to deal with staff, who have been subject to different training and to educational disciplines belonging to different professional bodies. He may have some degree of managerial skill and yet be ineffective when faced with the confusing array of pathologist, biochemist and technician as well as office girl, porter and domestic. It is important for senior staff to understand a little of their own attitudes and behaviour as well as those of their subordinates and superiors. Brown (1954) has stressed: 'We cannot understand the attitude of workers or management of workers unless they are seen in a historical context and unless it is realized that much that has been regarded as human nature is in fact purely the product of a particular culture at a particular stage of its development'.

Few observers can fail to notice a growing gap between the aims and ambitions of the professional groups and the needs of pathology departments. The professional bodies are doing what they were designed to do in protecting the interests of their members, it is true, but as the hospital service is the main employer and capable of setting its own standards the presence of professional bodies makes tactful administration imperative. It is the familiar situation of professional standards clashing with what the service can afford or requires. The three professional groups tend to assume what is best for them is also best for the clinicians who use the main services. The College of Pathology feels that the training of pathologists should override the short-term needs of departments as they stress in the Report of a Standing Committee of the College of Pathologists (1966d). The Institute increases the educational level of its courses to increase the status of technicians (*see* Report, I.M.L.T., 1965). These ambitions are pursued regardless of the financial situation of the N.H.S. and of what the hospital service can afford to allocate to diagnostic services.

Again the gap between the professional groups themselves is growing. Pathologists appear to present a unified front to the world at large but it is common to find that a team of pathologists working in the same group of hospitals or in laboratories of the same department are anything but united. The gap between technicians and pathologists is alarmingly wide and has increased since the President of the A.C.P. drew attention to it (Davey, 1954). Though the College of Pathology and the Institute may publicly say all is well between them this is not so in many departments. Pathologists, unable to control technicians as in the old days, are now calling for legislation to solve problems (for example, to make on-call duty a compulsory condition of service); at one stage during some salary negotiations they even recommended that a technician's annual increment should first have the approval of his pathology. There remains also a surprising and widening gap

27

in 1969 between technicians and their Institute; 5 per cent of members attended the 1960 Annual General Meeting and only 17 per cent bothered to vote for council members in the same year. Biochemists in District General Hospitals are often not accepted by pathologists or doctors as colleagues (Crichton, 1963), yet feel themselves to be something better than technicians. In some cases it is a question of status. Whitehead (1967) writes: 'It is felt that if good science graduates are to be encouraged into laboratories then regard will have to be paid to their status'.

THE DEVELOPMENT OF MEDICINE AND PATHOLOGY

By the second half of the nineteenth century medicine had organized itself into two main streams: the London Voluntary Hospitals with their medical schools; and the provincial Universities, which included a medical faculty. Several chairs of pathology had been established in the provincial Universities. Their pathology departments were almost entirely devoted to research and the teaching of histopathology, little diagnostic work being done. Both Cambridge and Glasgow were training technicians by the end of the century and three of these men—Norman, Mitchell and Mclean—were to play a major part in creating the Pathology and Bacteriology Assistants Association a few years later.

The situation in London developed in quite a different way. Here medicine was controlled by the great voluntary hospitals with their medical schools but had little connection with Universities apart from University College Hospital. These hospitals and medical schools were dominated by honorary physicians and surgeons who derived their income from private practice. They made great contributions to pathology as part of their work but did not see the need for pathologists as a separate body and in any case there was insufficient private practice in pathology to support an honorary pathologist. Pathology developed in London as an ancillary to medicine rather than as a subject on its own, a state of affairs which persisted until around 1930. The honorary surgeons and physicians in London were also the leaders of the two colleges —The Royal College of Physicians and the Royal College of Surgeons—and had great power in the world of medicine.

DEVELOPMENT OF PATHOLOGISTS

Before about 1880 the nearest approach to a laboratory was a microscope room where clinicians examined specimens such as blood and urine. The rather grudging acceptance of bacteriology as a science made it necessary for clinicians to provide better facilities and to delegate the technical work to another doctor whom they seemed to regard in consequence as an inferior. Foster, in 1961, wrote:

> The proud physician frankly considered the laboratory doctor beneath him and was most reluctant to admit him to equal consultation. It must however be admitted that the extravagant claims, the rapacity and arrogance of some bacteriologists did much to alienate even those physicians who were most appreciative of the possibilities of the laboratory in clinical medicine.

Evidence of this attitude still seems to exist today (Cappell, 1960). The bacteriologist was also expected to undertake any haematology and histology tests that were required. It was not considered to be a career in itself, however, and many physicians, even as late as the 1920s, felt that a few years spent in a laboratory were part of a physician's training.

The Pathology Society was formed in 1906 (Dible, 1957), to provide a learned society for doctors working in pathology and bacteriology, neither haematology nor biochemistry being sufficiently developed at this time to warrant separate mention. Support for the society came mainly from Scotland and the provinces, partly because of the attitude of the honorary clinicians in London, and partly because a London Pathology Society had been flourishing for some time. The journal of the Pathology Society was first published in 1907.

The society grew steadily and many wished to restrict membership as it grew larger and more difficult to run. Several unsuccessful attempts were made to divide the society into two parts one for pathology and one for bacteriology but this was a constant source of friction. Some members tried on several occasions to use the Society as a pressure group but the majority always refused, and it was this unwillingness to enter into medical politics that led pathologists in the provinces to form the Association of Clinical Pathologists in 1927.

The London voluntary hospitals were only slowly creating laboratories by the end of the nineteenth century, but the provincial voluntary hospitals developed theirs even more slowly. Wolverhampton and Swansea hospitals had laboratories by 1920 but there were very few others. These provincial hospitals were dependent

29

on public donations for their funds and little could be spared for a laboratory or a pathologist. Those who took posts in these hospitals had to eke out their low salaries by undertaking private work from outside their hospital. They were also dependent on the good will of the honorary staff for sending them work and passing on a part or all of the fee. Because they were paid a salary, provincial pathologists were usually barred from sitting on the hospital committee with the honorary physicians and surgeons.

Changes in the Organization of Hospitals

The introduction of bacteriology made it necessary for local authority medical officers of health to establish their own bacteriology laboratories to help them to control infectious diseases. These laboratories were at first set up in psychiatric and fever hospitals or as separate establishments in towns, but later as the local authorities took over poor law institutes and became responsible for running general hospitals the laboratories were developed in them. The most famous of these authorities was the London County Council who ran their hospitals most effectively under the direction of a chief medical officer on a group basis. A Group laboratory would serve a number of hospitals in the surrounding district, and each of these was expected to specialize in one or two lines of research and to act as a reference laboratory for the rest and also to train staff in techniques to their speciality. Technical staff had a grading system and the London County Council organized their own examination system. Day-release for students was established in 1946. Supplies were organized centrally from the Southern Group Laboratory—so successfully that it supplied many other organizations during the war and after the N.H.S. was created. A wide range of scientific journals were purchased and circulated round all laboratories, each being responsible for filing one or two of them.

By 1926 local authority laboratories were planning to accept pathology requests from any one. This alarmed provincial pathologists who looked on private practice as part of their income, so that: 'they saw the move as a definite threat to the whole future development of such a service in a clinical pathology centre, as it should be upon the (voluntary) hospital' (Foster, 1961).

Formation of the Association of Clinical Pathologists

As the Pathology Society was opposed to behaving as any sort of pressure group, pathologists led by S. C. Dyke formed the Association of Clinical Pathology (A.C.P.) with the objects of improving the standards and teaching of pathology; improving the status of pathologists so to ensure their having the same standing as consultants; and securing adequate remuneration for hospital pathologists. A group of Clinical Pathologists was formed within the British Medical Association and a resolution was passed at the A.G.M. of 1927 stating that fees for private pathology work should be the property of the pathologist. Dyke considered this resolution to be the 'Magna Carta' of Clinical Pathology. The A.C.P. persuaded the University of London to institute a Diploma in Clinical Pathology but this never became popular. The A.C.P. expended most of its energies on improving the pay and status of pathologists up to 1939, by which time 'most pathologists were in administrative charge of a busy department' (Stevens, 1966).

As the prospects of war increased in 1939, steps were taken to organize hospitals on an area basis and the Emergency Medical Service was created and included pathology departments. At about the same time the Public Health Laboratory Service (P.H.L.S.) was created to assist local authority laboratories in providing a bacteriology service which would cover the whole of the country and also help in the event of epidemics in war time. An embryonic Blood Transfusion Service was organized using the existing arrangements already made on a voluntary basis by some pathology departments.

It became apparent during the organization of the E.M.S. service that something more permanent would have to be created to replace the existing mixture of voluntary and local authority hospitals. Many schemes were proposed for organizing hospitals and among them was the concept of Regionalization of Pathology (Dyke, 1940).

Dyke stressed that pathology services were badly organized because provincial voluntary hospitals were short of money, though they did their best. He pointed out that these departments had tried to make money and had the local authorities supported them by sending them work instead of using their own laboratories, pathology services would have flourished. Dyke proposed two services; the public health service and a clinical pathology laboratory service run on the lines of the London County Council scheme. He advocated that pathologists should be allowed private practice and that technicians should have proper salary scales. He saw the pathology service flourishing if departments in existing voluntary hospitals could be adequately financed.

31

When the Health Service finally came into existence both local authority and voluntary hospitals were taken over and only the teaching hospitals were organized separately. Pathology departments in both local authority and voluntary hospitals were gradually expanded being organized within groups of hospitals under management committees who were responsible for the day-to-day running of their hospitals and, of course, their laboratories. The groups were organized into regions under the direction of Regional Hospital Boards who were responsible to the Minister of Health. The majority of pathologists became consultants and, as such, were employed by Regional Boards; technicians on the other hand were employed by the relevant H.M.C. A Regional Pathology Advisory Committee was formed to advise the regional boards and a Central Pathology Advisory Committee—with one member from each region and representative of the teaching school—to advise the Minister on the laboratory Service.

The P.H.L.S. was not included in the Health Service until after 1960 and in the interim was run by the Medical Research Council for the Ministry. This service is an excellent example of the benefits and limitations of a system which combines central control and co-ordination, with adequate delegation of authority to directors of individual laboratories. The P.H.L.S. set up a good system of reference laboratories; provided reagents which could not be obtained commercially; provided expert advice; published a bulletin covering both techniques and views; and now circulates a wide range of scientific journals. Yet today it is not considered by some technicians to be a happy service to work for.

Similar to the P.H.L.S. is the Blood Transfusion Service which was loosely organized on a regional basis by the end of the war. Regional Hospital Boards took over responsibility and provided finance for the transfusion service in their region. The director of each regional laboratory sat on the national committee which set technical standards, and decided on research projects. However, this division between financial responsibility resting with the Board and decisions on research being taken by the national committee, induces a feeling of frustration among staff since Regional Boards are more likely to finance the research they consider worthwhile or that which looks like being successful.

These two services provide a sharp contrast with pathology departments in Hospitals. Here pathologists are employed by Regional Boards; the H.M.C. employs biochemists and technicians and finances pathology departments. Regional pathology advisory committees have never been successful in co-ordinating pathology departments within their region. The Central Advisory Committee has not exercised a strong and co-ordinating function and in result the development is taking place in a piecemeal fashion.

The Need for a Higher Qualification

Although the great majority of pathologists in posts in 1948 became consultants on the creation of the N.H.S. this did not appear to solve the problems of status. They were very conscious of the lack of a suitable qualification and were also aware of their lack of power in medical politics compared with surgeons or physicians each with the backing of their Royal College. Discussions on possible remedies took place in 1953 among members of the A.C.P. and the Pathology Society about the M.R.C.P. The Royal College of Physicians was willing to establish a Mastership in Clinical Pathology but this would not enable the holder to be elected to F.R.C.P. Pathologists were sharply divided among themselves about the formation of a College of Pathology and the division appeared to be between the old pathologist who had qualified pre-war (the majority of whom were working in London), and the new post-war generation of pathologists who worked in the main in the provinces. The R.C.P. later improved its offer and agreed to set up a Faculty of Pathology to be run by pathologists themselves. By this time those pathologists in favour of forming a College of their own had a small majority. After ten years of discussion the College of Pathology was formed in 1962 and grew rapidly. Until 1966 all pathologists of consultant status were eligible for membership without examination. There was a brief but sharp discussion as to whether non-medical workers, such as biochemists, could be eligible for membership but as it turned out biochemists did not want to join.

The first examinations of the College of Pathology were held in 1964 in two parts: the first a broadly-based examination after two years' full-time work in a pathology department and, after a further three years' full-time work, the second and final examination in one of the four main branches; haematology, biochemistry, pathology or bacteriology. Pass rates in the first examination were disappointing, and in 1965, 45 passed out of 124 candidates—this probably because of the poor training which housemen and registrars received while working in pathology departments. An editorial comment in the *Lancet* July 9th 1966, expressed the view that the College was in a position to insist that the needs of trainee

33

Pathologists be considered before the short-term needs of the laboratory so that, with skilful management, a valuable lever could be constructed with which to raise standards, in space, staff and equipment of many laboratories. Yet management seems to be the one subject that neither the College nor the A.C.P. feels it necessary to teach its members.

The position regarding the training of pathologists today is that the College of Pathology seems to be teaching trainee pathologists technology so that they can supervise and control the work of technicians. The feeling that a pathologist must know techniques if he is to supervise technicians, is still strong. The College wanted the first training period to be general in content, and the second to specialize in one discipline but after a few years they reduced the range of the primary examination from four to two subjects. The trainee pathologist thus has a great burden of learning in that—after obtaining his medical qualification—he then has to start on a vast new field of scientific knowledge instead of practising medicine as other clinicians do. By the time he becomes a senior registrar, particularly if he is not in a teaching hospital department, routine work takes most of his time, leaving little time for study. As a consultant the demands on his time—particularly if he is the senior or group consultant—are great because of consultations with clinicians, administrative work and post mortems and it becomes a herculean task to keep abreast of the new ideas which are flooding into his department. On the other hand if he becomes a consultant pathologist in charge of a laboratory he may have difficulty in adequately filling his working day and may well undertake technical work in order to do this.

The persistence of The College, in insisting that trainee pathologists learn so much technique, is strange in view of the fact that much of a consultant's time is spent on such vital but mundane matters as getting money from his group secretary or from the regional senior administrative officer and providing factual evidence to support his claim for such money; or dealing with the enthusiastic clinician who wants obscure tests carried out on some of his patients; or dealing with the minor problems that arise in his department. All these jobs could be done with less effort and more success if some training in managerial skills was given.

Consultant Pathologists in General Hospitals

Turning from a consideration of the development of pathologists as professionals it is relevant to ask how they have been developing within their own departments. With the creation of the N.H.S. pathologists became consultants, being employed by regional boards and being responsible to the Senior Administrative Medical Officer. Their contract on full time or part time made them responsible for running the pathology department for an H.M.C. but it does not lay down how they should spend their time or divide it between hospital and private work.

For the first few years of the N.H.S., life for the average hospital pathologist was pleasant. Clinicians had overcome their prejudices of the 1930s and accepted the pathology department as making a useful contribution to medicine. The work itself was increasing slowly but the pace of the department was not altering very much. The range of tests was still small enough for one man to carry all the normal values and the significance of abnormal values in his head and in fact be the all-round expert; opinions were still valuable. Much of the work was related to a diagnosis. By the 1950s changes in medical and surgical practice were reflected plainly in the department. As Stevens (1966) says:

> The patient was no longer admitted into nursing care while awaiting the weekly visit of the great man (consultant). Instead the junior doctor sprang immediately into action, armed with modern therapeutic drugs and access to refined pathological and radiological diagnostic facilities.

The great increase in requests which resulted from this change came at a time when money was becoming scarce in the N.H.S. Some pathologists, particularly those supervising all four laboratories in their department, were content to retreat into histopathology and post mortems and to hand over the rest of the technical work to technicians. Others resented their growing dependence on technicians, feeling that as Davey (1954) said:

> The man (pathologist) who does not know about technique will we unable to detect the errors and short cuts that tend to creep into our work. He is then at the mercy of the technician who is not usually slow to appreciate the fact.

From 1955 to 1967 work has increased, money is now very short and technology too varied and complex to be grasped by one man. Automatic equipment seemed to offer a way out of the problems arriving in the wake of increased work, but although much automated equipment has been purchased the problems still exist. Pathology departments are having to function faster simply to maintain their present position. Some pathologists have passed over more work to technicians and biochemists, some have even given up signing reports (often regarded as the last vestige of authority) and some have opted out of administering their departments to a large extent. Professor Cappell (1960) summarized pathologists' feelings.

> Colleagues have expressed anxiety on this score (increasing work) and deprecate the almost total submergence of the clinical pathologist in carrying out the routine work test at the behest of the clinicians, a position which may well induce a feeling of inferiority if the pathologist has no say in the selection of work he has to do, and allows himself to be used as one whose work is merely ancillary to that of the clinician . . . The medical and technical staff of hospital pathology departments has all too often been kept at so low a level that energies are wholly spent in getting through the day's work and this is all the more true when the duties involve so-called emergency calls at night and at week-ends, not all of which are real emergencies.

Pathologists have had consultant grade and pay for 20 years now; they also have their own college and higher qualifications and it would be reasonable to assume that they would be satisfied but this does not seem to be the case. However when a comparison is made between the idealistic concept of the post of consultant pathologist and reality it is easy to understand.

The pathologist has been through a system of medical education designed to produce clinicians who behave in an authoritarian way, as individualists, with the expectancy of becoming consultants. The archetype pathologist is based on the professor of pathology who in his own department has absolute authority, equality with other professors, responsibility for research and teaching and is not burdened with routine work for other clinicians of lower rank than himself. Pathologists probably see their job as primarily concerned with research and—only a poor second, as being a technical service for clinicians carried out by a large group of skilled, willing and unquestioning assistants. And all this possibly combined with the advantages of a private practice. Cappell (1960) stresses: 'It was not so long ago that the pathology department was known as the research department'.

This picture is in marked contrast to the reality in which a pathologist is the administrative head of a busy department and is responsible—as are the heads of other hospital departments—to the H.M.C. for organizing the pathology service. The department is too large for the pathologist to supervise all the work so he has to delegate some or all of it to technicians who as a group have skill, ambitions of their own, control of their professional affairs and who will leave to go to a better job. As departments become larger the more difficult it is to run them on authoritarian lines. The transition from a small department with one pathologist and one chief technician, to a large department with several pathologists and several chief technicians presents sociological and organizational problems. Technicians are beginning to see their department as providing a service for clinicians rather than as supporting a pathologist as a consultant. Clinicians are sending in more work than a pathology department can comfortably manage but the pathologist does not know how to stop them without damaging his image and hence decreasing his status or challenging the idea of that clinical freedom so dear to him. Again, clinicians now want more tests to provide factual information and seem to be less interested in consulting pathologists for their opinion. Again, the biochemists in the department are beginning to speak a language no longer intelligible to many pathologists.

In the face of all these difficulties which pathologists face each day, the aims and ambitions of their professional bodies seem abstract. Over the course of years pathologists have had to create different bodies to meet the needs of the moment; first the Pathology Society—a learned society; then the Association of Clinical Pathology concerning itself with a mixture of medical politics, matters of status and pathology; and finally a College of Pathology to provide higher qualifications. Judging from their present difficulties the next body should be a faculty of departmental management and business studies.

THE DEVELOPMENT OF TECHNICIANS

Technicians were first employed as unskilled laboratory assistants in pathology departments in teaching hospitals and universities. Their duties were largely menial and prospects were poor with little chance of advancement in spite of the gradual need for skilled help. After an abortive attempt by Mclean in 1896, Norman —a technician working in Manchester—began to organize the Pathology and Bacteriology Laboratory Assistants Association

(P.B.L.A.A.) with the help of other technicians such as Mitchell, Chopping and Mclean. Norman decided that a militant organization would be useless and that it was necessary rather to create one which would strengthen trust between employer and employee. The purpose of the Association was to enable laboratory assistants to meet and exchange ideas; also to supply information about appointments. The first meetings took place in 1912 and from then on the Association developed. The first rebuff to the organization came when they tried to convince the Royal Army Medical Corps of the value of experienced laboratory assistants and were told that these laboratory assistants were considered to be unskilled menials (Mitchell, 1933). This showed the need for a system of examination and qualifications. Classes were started in one or two places in 1920 on an informal basis and developed into regular weekly courses in hospital laboratories. With the help of members of the Pathology Society examinations were held in 1929 and the first Intermediate examination in 1936.

Norman also initiated the Journal of the Association in 1913 which included editorial comment, contributions of original scientific articles and abstracts from scientific journals. Though the journal appeared rather irregularly it was of great importance in forming a link between members. A monthly bulletin with news and reports of Council activities and vacancies was brought out in 1934. The first conference, modelled on the meeting of the Pathology Society, was held in Edinburgh in 1924. This was a great success and many more have followed. Today this function, now a triennial affair, is the most successful function of the Institute. All these activities represented a great achievement by this small group of assistants led by Norman, and laid the foundation for technicians of an effective professional body. By the mid-thirties the Association had grown to several hundred members with probably the majority of technicians working in hospitals, and the Council considered that some sort of legal status was required. This could be achieved in a number of ways and it was agreed in 1938, though not unanimously, to form an institute in the form of a limited company.

Events were now overtaken by the war and the P.B.L.A.A. helped technicians within the Emergency Hospital Service. The Association showed little interest in ideas that were being expressed and widely discussed about the formation of a health service. It was only noted with regret that the Association had not been invited to express a view on the plans for such a service.

About this time there was a strong move from members to get the Association to act as a trade union. However council resisted the request as it preferred to rely on the good offices of the Pathology Society. This was surprising in view of the fact that pathologists had found the Pathology Society unwilling to act as any sort of pressure group and had formed the A.C.P. in consequence.

The Formation of the Institute of Medical Laboratory Technology

Negotiations for forming a limited company, which specifically excluded trade union activities, were completed in 1942 and the first council meeting held in 1943. This year was full of activity; a board of examiners was set up with members from the Institute and the Pathology Society and a system of Intermediate and final examination was devised; school certificate was laid down as the entry requirement; and finally members from the P.B.L.A.A. were given until October 31st of that year to transfer to the Institute—after this date entry was to be by examination only. It is difficult to understand why this action in regard to the date of transfer was taken so rapidly when many technicians were still in the armed forces—though possibly it was similar to the situation in 1918: 'As war conditions developed a new danger became apparent, for it seemed that, at the end of the war, there would be an influx of war trained men and women into laboratory life. . . ' (Mitchell, 1933). On returning from war service a number of technicians found themselves faced with an examination to become an associate of the Institute or barred from the post of technician as the Associateship was now a condition of service in many hospitals. Some changed their job, some found jobs as technicians in out-of-the-way places and some joined the Association of Scientific Workers, a union catering for technicians and functioning as a sort of unofficial opposition.

By the late 1940s, the Council of the Institute had every reason to feel satisfied with themselves as they had achieved every major ambition of the founder members. The Institute's qualifications had been accepted as a condition of employment for technicians in the N.H.S. and were much sought after in Commonwealth Countries. Training courses had become firmly established in most parts of the country in the form of evening classes held in hospital laboratories. The Journal and the Gazette were on a sound footing and membership was steadily increasing. The only failure was that the Institute had been unable to gain a place on the staff side of the Whitley Council. The senior members of the Council saw

39

no reason to change their paternal attitude to members or their traditionally acquiescent one to pathologists.

Trade Unions

At this point it is appropriate to explain the organization and function of the Whitley Council in the National Health Service. The four trade unions with technicians in membership in 1947 were invited to form the staff side of committee 'A' of the Professional and Technical Division 'B' of the General Whitley Council or to give it its more familiar name P.T.B. 'A'. The unions were: the Association of Scientific Workers (now amalgamated in the Association of Scientific, Technical and Managerial Staffs) and with the largest membership; the National Union of Public Employees; the Confederation of Health Service Employees; and the National and Local Government Officers Association—since 1955, with the Institute (I.M.L.T.) as advisers. The management side of P.T.B. 'A' is composed of representatives of the Ministry of Health, Boards of Governors of teaching hospitals, Regional Hospitals Boards, Association of Hospital Management Committees and the Boards of Management (Scotland). The Treasury is not represented but their presence is always felt. At the height of militant trade unionism among technicians in 1961 only 50 per cent actually belonged to any union.

The General Council draws up basic conditions of service concerning such matters as hours of work and holidays. The P.T.B. 'A' draws up regulations concerning rates of pay, grades and the 'on-call' service. The four unions of the staff side conduct their business with skill and it is unusual for any serious disagreement to occur between them. Inevitably there was and still is a certain amount of inter-union rivalry as well as a tendency to adopt a threatening or aggressive attitude to the management side in order to encourage or impress members. Negotiations have been bedevilled by the influence of the Treasury over salaries and several times unions have been forced to go to arbitration over wage claims. It is disappointing that none of the unions have sought to improve their capacity for competing with the management side by collecting and analysing facts. Until recently the staff side did not know how many pathology departments existed in the N.H.S. or how many technicians were employed in each grade. It is generally thought that it was the negotiating skill of the unions which won the major salary increase of 30 per cent in 1962 during the first pay pause. It was more likely that the Treasury were taken aback at the number of qualified technicians who left the service in 1962—63 as the total number in the N.H.S. decreased by 390 at that time, compared with the average annual increase of 75 (*see* Table 6 on page 19). In such matters the management does not appear to be any better informed than the staff side.

For the Institute (I.M.L.T.), in its hour of great achievement, events began to take place such as a rapid increase in a membership having new ambitions and changes, too, in technical education, bringing about a new situation which the Council failed to detect or appreciate. Conditions were difficult when the Institute was first formed for travel was restricted and expensive and so of necessity the organization had to be centralized, and easy and inexpensive to run. The General Purposes Committee was given executive power to be exercised as and when demanded (Report, I.M.L.T., 1947). The Council consisted of both a regionally and a nationally elected membership. The new members joining the Institute after the war tended to see it solely as an examining body. They were interested in obtaining a qualification in order to get a job and were prepared to move to get a good one. By the mid-fifties this post-war group began to want some say in the control of the profession they followed for they felt the need for an improved status in keeping with their growing expertise and responsibilities. Council took little notice of these demands considering them to be a little irresponsible and, in consequence, making no move to recognize the structure of the Institute to make it more democratic or to encourage members to feel that they had any say in their own affairs.

The gap so created between senior Council members and the post-war group widened beyond all expectation and by 1960 only 56 out of 8,250 members attended the Annual General Meeting and less than 20 per cent voted to elect council members. In 1967 this situation had not altered as only 80 out of a total of 13,670 members attended the A.G.M. Members wanted an election address from prospective Council members instead of merely a list of names, many of which were unknown to them. Moreover five out of a total of seven members of the General Purposes Committee were unchanged for more than ten years. Matters came to a head at the 1961 A.G.M. when Council proposed a motion to double the existing fees for the final examination from £5 to £10. The proposition was heavily defeated mainly by proxy votes, which were considered by Council to be part of a deliberately organized campaign; this they denounced in such phrases as 'alien', 'irresponsible', 'nothing to do with democracy' (Report I.M.L.T. Gazette, July 1963). They did not try to see the underlying reasons for this action. In 1963 the same motion was carried at a meeting by 214 votes to 32 out of a total membership of 8,000. It hardly seemed like democracy or responsible leadership when less than 3 per cent of the membership voted. However following the defeat of 1961, Council chairman admitted that contact with members was difficult and public relations were not Council's strong point but at the same time he felt that the opposition among members was not serious. The conflict between Council and members is inevitable but has advantages in that it helps to maintain commitment and emotional involvement of members in the affairs of the profession, and encourages the free interplay of contending interests.

The Need for Higher Qualifications

In 1964, in an effort to increase the status of its examinations, Council introduced an advanced examination open to Associates only. Fellows of the Institute felt this gave the Associate a great advantage when applying for senior jobs but nevertheless Council insisted on the restriction. In 1966 Council introduced the idea of a graduate membership for those taking a degree level examination after obtaining a Higher National Certificate in Medical Laboratory Sciences; this was to be awarded for the first time in 1971. Any existing Fellows would have to pass the H.N.C. before being allowed to sit for the examination leading to Graduate Membership. This was an attempt by Council to retain control over the profession but virtually at the cost of cutting off existing Fellows from a chance of becoming graduate members. The postwar technician needed the Institute as there was then and still is no one at hospital or Regional Board level who looks after their interests or provides understanding and support. Hospital secretaries usually restrict their interest to the conditions of service and many pathologists were not well disposed towards technicians during the 1950s; indeed only a small minority of pathologists took any interest in technicians affairs until the last few years.

This lack of understanding, between Council and members, influenced Council's actions in a number of ways causing even more frustration among members. Norman, being chairman of Council, was a member of the Cope Committee which recommended state registration for medical auxiliaries, as they were then called. He was also a member of a working party on the draft of the Professions Supplementary to Medicine Bill, which led to the formation of the Registration Board in 1968; he must therefore have realized the full implications of the Bill. Yet in 1954 after several years of discussion Council was not in a position to offer an opinion on state registration. They finally decided to co-operate in formulating the Bill on the advice of their solicitors but not of their members (I.M.L.T. Annual Report, 1958). Both Council and members became much more concerned about the cost and mechanics of registration than about the purpose of the Bill which could give members control over their own profession. The Institute had been virtually powerless to enforce minimum standards in pathology departments and technical colleges with regard to training student technicians and the Bill would give them power to enforce such standards. Immediately before it was published, Council worked hard and succeeded in obtaining a majority of technicians on the registration instead of doctors—a crucial point. The Bill went through its first and second reading in 1959 before most technicians had realized what was happening; it was finally passed in 1960 and then and only then did Council appear to make an all-out effort to persuade members of the value of the act.

Another example of Council misinterpreting the needs of the situation was in its efforts to behave as a trade union. In 1945 prior to the institution of the N.H.S. there were three different salary scales for technicians employed in hospital laboratories; this caused many anomalies. It was clear that someone had to co-ordinate or simplify these scales and that this was a job for a trade union. Instead of accepting its limitations in such matters and advising members to join a trade union, Council spent the next ten years behaving like a trade union itself, and only being admitted to the staff side as advisers after a long dispute with the trade unions representing technicians. Failure to accept reality and appreciate the wider role of trade unions led Council to miss the opportunity of making a unique contribution to the Whitley Council in general and to the problems of technicians in particular.

One very influential factor in framing the policy of Council since 1945 is that Norman and many other early workers in the P.B.L.A.A. spent the greater part of their working life outside hospitals, in university departments, research units or veterinary laboratories. Norman worked at the Animal Research Institute in Weybridge from 1913—immediately after he formed the Institute—until he retired and he thus dominated Council's thinking for nearly 50 years. In the formative years of the Institute, this lack of hospital experience made little difference but it certainly slowed up the progress of the Institute after 1947. Chief technicians have long felt the need to express a collective point of view on matters concerning pathology departments but the Institute will not accept or encourage this role. The vacuum is now being filled at regional hospital board level by chief technicians meeting on a formal or informal basis to discuss matters of common interest as departmental managers.

The development of technicians within laboratories has been influenced both by the quantity of the work and the changes in technology. The first technicians were skilled craftsmen working at the beginning of the century under the close supervision of a pathologist or a research worker—a simple, straightforward master-and-servant relationship. Then, a pathologist would have one or two assistants working under him and the contact was direct with no problems of communication or of supervision and with obvious and accepted differences in status. The pattern of the work altered at a leisurely pace over the next few decades and changes were easily assimilated by technicians. Existing equipment was also developed at much the same sort of pace with little new being introduced. This broad leisurely development of technology brought about few changes in the situation of technicians within their laboratories until a number of events coincided in the late 1940s.

As the N.H.S. settled down, the demand for laboratory services began to increase, a new generation of technicians was recruited and many new ideas were introduced in consequence. These recruits were well trained under the new system and so were able to cope with the new techniques and equipment that were being introduced. They were eager to learn both the techniques and the theory behind them. As the number of requests for diagnostic tests rose, technicians were given increasing responsibility for the technical work since some pathologists were now being overwhelmed by the routine work.

The Effects of Advances in Technology

Until about 1948 the bacteriology laboratory was considered to be the centre of the pathology department with the chief technician, not greatly encumbered by administrative duties, generally in charge. With the advent of antibiotics the role of this laboratory declined in general hospitals. It is interesting to speculate as to whether clinicians would have used antibiotics with more care if pathologists had seen their function in a different light—as being rather that of adviser to clinicians than as consultant. As bacteriology work began to level off, that in haematology began to expand. More clinicians required more haematological information as anaemias were better understood and classified in scientific terms and vitamin B_{12} was discovered and used for treatment. For a time the haematology laboratory became the hub of the department, orientated to patients, carrying out relatively simple estimations and techniques. Within a few years as biochemistry branched off and became a separate subject from medical physiology, it in turn began to appear as the dominating discipline in pathology departments. This branching-off process was accelerated by major discoveries in technology, such as flame photometry, which simplified the estimation of blood electrolytes; electrophoresis which opened up the analysis of serum proteins; and chromatography which gave new scope to the indentification and estimation of complex biological substances. The technicians tended to become involved and increasingly preoccupied with techniques and equipment and less concerned with patients and there was a growing tendency to attract newly qualified technicians with their greater knowledge of science. In both haematology and biochemistry laboratories the number of requests has increased, but biochemistry laboratories have in addition increased their range of routine tests from approximately 10 to 30. They have enthusiastically welcomed automated and electronic equipment in consequence.

The histology laboratory has altered least of all. The methods of preparing histological sections for pathologists—its main job—reflect the conservative approach of pathologists who still prefer standard, well-tried methods which have not changed much since the beginning of the century. The processing of tissue has been automated but little else. The histology laboratory, then, in District General Hospitals, with its unhurried approach and limited technology has tended to attract technicians who do not like the bustle or contact with patients often obtaining in haematology laboratories or the more high-powered technology called for in biochemistry; because of this too, such laboratories may have tended to collect the unambitious technicians.

By the end of the 1950s, as technicians took over greater responsibility for routine work which by now was less concerned with diagnosis, they began to look to the clinician with his need for information rather than to the pathologist. To understand and cope with new advances in technology, technicians were compelled to learn much new theory but at the same time some pathologists appeared to take less interest in new methods and to make a little less effort to absorb new ideas and developments as they arrived in the laboratory: for example, coagulation defects, auto-immune diseases and enzymology. At this stage, technicians were specializing to a marked degree and felt inhibited by the need to pass a final examination in a second subject which held little interest for them. As technicians matured and began to take charge of a laboratory they tended to behave more like technologists, looking for new techniques, modifying old ones. They also began to take decisions themselves on how to produce the information that clinicians require—which test to use and when to use a screening test rather than a complex test. Furthermore, they acquired considerable skill in supervising other technicians, organizing work and training students.

Technicians originally undertook emergency duties on a voluntary basis, feeling they were contributing to the good of the patient. As emergency work increased a system of payment was introduced which incidentally compensated for the very low salaries in the same way as does overtime in a factory or payment for domiciliary visits by pathologists. However by the early 1960s doctors were using the emergency service less for the benefit of the patient and rather more for their own convenience and even occasionally for their protection and it was becoming, in effect, a 24-hour service. Trainee pathologists who undertook emergency work also felt indignant about the attitude of housemen who sent in such work, feeling that 'they treated us like mere technicians' (Walsh, 1967). Many experienced technicians with years of service felt equally strongly about the situation and stopped doing 'on-call' duties altogether; indeed the complaints about payment for 'on-call' duties were in many cases a symptom of an underlying dissatisfaction. Pathologists misinterpreted the situation and tried to make participation in the emergency service a condition of employment but were unsuccessful.

Technicians were working harder in 1960 than ever before and carrying greater responsibilities. They resented their low salaries and the fact that at that time training of staff had been subordinated to routine work. There was talk of strikes and demonstrations were held but not until they had demonstrated their dissatisfaction by leaving the N.H.S. in large numbers in 1962–63 did they manage to get a pay increase. In the middle of the pay pause in 1961 they were awarded a 30 per cent increase and between 1962 and 1966 average increases of 4, 7, 13 and 3 per cent were given.

The pressure of work had built up by 1965 and pathology departments became very large, some with over 60 technicians and several pathologists. Chief technicians began to develop into departmental managers concerned with sharing out money and resources, co-ordinating laboratories, recruiting staff, and generally becoming less involved with technology. Automation had been introduced a few years earlier and had been welcomed enthusiastically by most technicians although some of the older ones were a little apprehensive. However, after a few years' experience many chief technicians began to temper their enthusiasm about complex automated equipment particularly in small and medium size pathology departments.

Now, as departmental managers they are encountering problems calling for a different approach and new techniques such as forward planning, cost-effectiveness and manpower planning. They are beginning to face pressure for an extended working day in order to keep automated equipment in full use while knowing that many clinicians cannot use more information. Chief technicians in large departments have been sandwiched between the senior consultant pathologist in charge of the department and other consultant pathologists in charge of laboratories and are now beginning to learn how to cope with this situation. They have had contact with hospital administrative staff and are beginning to develop skills in administrative matters and have found technological training—which stresses the importance of a process of analytical thought leading to a decision—a useful asset in this situation.

In the 20 years or so since the beginning of the N.H.S. technicians have developed into the most powerful and successful group of the Professions Supplementary to Medicine. Their salary scale is now the envy of other professional and technical groups. Administrators regard them with a mixture of pride and horror and pathologists are no longer sure what to make of their erstwhile assistants. Their educational system will be a model for many other groups in the N.H.S. and has provided technical colleges with a challenge in the field of education.

Many chief technicians are no longer struggling against pathologists as they tended to do in the mid-1950s but rather, at last,

47

coming to terms with them. Until recently they did not want to stop being technicians, giving up the skill they had spent years acquiring and the status this skill and their qualifications brought them among their fellow technicians. A serious problem faces the experienced technician who, graded as chief I, is in charge of a laboratory but doing relatively little administration and engaged in the more complex technology. To gain more money and higher status he must be promoted to the grade of chief technician II and undertake mainly administrative work, giving up the technology which he enjoyed. Once he has taken the decision to become a chief II and takes up his new post he will find the job confusing because it has never been clearly described to him. No one will explain the difference between being technically in charge of his department and supervising his senior staff in their technical work. If he does not receive support from his pathologists he will tend to end up with such jobs as ordering stores, drawing up holiday lists and supervising the domestic staff. Alternatively he may retreat away from this difficult situation, placing the onus on his pathologist. This is seeing his job in a limited role for in fact the staff are dependent on him to keep the pathologist informed on the staff's point of view and on what is going on in the department. If the chief technician opts out of this—as commonly happens— he is cutting the staff off from the pathologist and forcing them to find alternative ways of getting their views across. It is possible that he will react to this difficult situation as many chiefs do and fight every inch of the way with his pathologist over each imagined or real slight. He will thus close the formal line of communication and cut off technicians completely again forcing them to find unofficial means of voicing their views and their needs. It is not enough to do the job of chief technician as he sees it himself for his staff also rely on his ability to carry out his function. He is forced to choose occasionally between protecting his dignity or keeping open the lines of communication with his pathologist and so maintaining a relationship with him that enables them to talk together honestly. A pathologist may alter some working arrangements in his department without consulting his chief technician; he will in fact be taking over the job of the chief technician for a short time, consciously or unconsciously. His chief technician is then faced with a choice of reacting adversely or ignoring the matter and in effect, retreating. Either action will tend to close the line of communication between them putting the technical staff at a considerable disadvantage. Whatever he does it will be absolutely obvious to his subordinates so the chief technician and pathologist need to understand what is happening and why.

THE DEVELOPMENT OF BIOCHEMISTS

Biochemistry was the last of the four subjects or disciplines to develop, consequently biochemists did not appear in pathology departments until after 1920 and then only in very small numbers. The impetus for their introduction came from the use of insulin in the treatment of diabetics requiring a large number of bloodsugar estimations. Before this period the range of biochemical tests was very small. The number of biochemists increased slowly and reached 211 in 1956 and 329 in 1965—a small number when compared with the number of pathology departments in the N.H.S. Before 1945, biochemists were employed only in the very large voluntary hospitals and a few of the larger local authority hospitals. There were also chemical pathologists who specialized in biochemistry though many had no specific qualifications in chemistry.

The biochemist runs his laboratory in collaboration with technicians and is responsible for the routine work as well as for developing new methods; he also undertakes research on his own initiative and at the request of the pathologist or clinicians. The normal qualification is an honours degree in chemistry or physiology or, more recently, in biochemistry. Graduates entering the service without an honours degree will be paid £100 per annum less. The salaries of biochemists are roughly the same as those of qualified technicians and it is only at the top of the senior biochemists scale that they are higher. Unfortunately university courses followed by graduate biochemists do not include the principles of analysis or instruments and are more concerned with theoretical than with applied biochemistry. The graduate enters pathology departments without any knowledge of hospitals, patients or doctors and has to learn after appointment many of the skills he requires—such as that of supervision.

The Need for Higher Qualifications

In common with pathologists and technicians, biochemists have felt the need for a higher qualification particularly for those seeking senior and principal posts. The Association of Biochemists and other interested bodies created a Mastership in Clinical Biochemistry (M.C.B.) with stringent training requirements which only a graduate working in or near a teaching hospital could fulfil. No doubt the M.C.B. will become a necessary qualification for senior and principal grades in future. This post-graduate training for a higher academic qualification may well have led biochemists to ignore the skills they need to use every day in supervising staff and organizing work. The Association of Clinical Biochemists recently complained that 20 per cent of basic grade biochemists were unsupervised by scientifically trained staff. Biochemists have a difficult position in pathology departments for having no medical qualification they are not accepted on equal terms by pathologists. On the other hand, being university graduates, they would not want to be classed with technicians. As a group, biochemists are orientated to technology and research rather than to service to clinicians because their training has emphasized research and tended to devalue applied knowledge. They accept without question the steady increase in the amount of work. With the expansion of biochemistry laboratories, biochemists are having to supervise large groups of staff and this is straining their ability as supervisors. They are seeking to solve their problems of increasing work-loads with automated equipment which is putting an even greater strain on their supervisory skill.

SUMMARY

The development of pathology has been influenced by scientific discoveries, by medical practice and by the maturing professional groups concerned. Pathologists have created three bodies to meet different needs as they arose. Technicians are now somewhat confused about their needs and the future of the Institute is uncertain. Biochemists have created a professional body including two types of professionals—those medically qualified and science graduates —and have yet to come to terms with the difficulties arising from this situation.

Changes have been considerably influenced by developments in technology for automated equipment not only simplifies the work but also brings changes in how departments are run as well as sociological changes among all grades of staff. Changes in medical practice—such as clinicians requiring large quantities of information not connected with diagnosis—are having their effect on pathology departments.

This review of the development of pathology and the professions shows that change does not generally take place rapidly. It often takes 15–20 years to find solutions and to introduce successful change—as with the formation of the College of Pathology. When change does take place rapidly (such as the change from a system of evening classes to block-release for training of technicians), many problems will appear—as opinions and attitudes will not have altered similarly fast. There are no examples of a new system wholly replacing an old one; changes are always evolutionary or adaptive, being moulded by the relative strength of the pressure groups involved. One lesson that can be learnt is that in order to have a higher chance of success changes that are evolutionary should be sought. Mistakes have been made because there were no adequate terms of reference or common understanding of the problems (for example, in the failure to make the A.C.P. a qualifying body in 1927). In order to find realistic terms of reference the problems must be clearly perceived and since medicine and technology are not static the terms of reference must be continually reviewed.

CHAPTER 3

DEPARTMENTAL MANAGEMENT

INTRODUCTION

Attempts to describe how to manage pathology departments will often founder because there are widely different views on their function or purpose. When asked to describe it technicians, biochemists and pathologists would all talk about a diagnostic service for the benefit of patients and then perhaps add a few words about the importance of research. Only a minority would include training technicians and an even smaller minority would mention training of biochemists and pathologists. This emphasis on the diagnostic service for patients may be due to the idea that the status of hospital staff depends on how directly they deal with patients for the highest status is given to consultant clinicians. This vague definition of purpose makes it difficult to teach anyone how to run a pathology department and also it makes it difficult to measure how efficiently it is being run or how effectively it is achieving its purpose. It may well account for the uncertainty and lack of sense of purpose that exists among all groups of staff in pathology departments today.

Accepting this usual definition for a moment, the job of the top team is to organize their department to provide a diagnostic service while they are also carrying out their consultative and technical work. They rarely if ever consider management to be an important part of their job and so many departments are managed by default or unconsciously. Departments tend to run themselves, changes being made in response to pressure rather than as a result of conscious planning. The general concept of the purpose of pathology departments seems to change from one situation to the next. Diagnosis of a patient's condition is a first essential but diagnosis of organizational problems in pathology departments is rare and they are treated symptomatically, the cause seldom being investigated. The effects of this symptomatic treatment on other hospital departments is ignored.

In these circumstances the struggle for personal status, ambition and empire building are all too common. Decisions are frequently based on power or personal status rather than on logic, planning, the needs of clinicians or even of patients. This attitude is demonstrated by the pathologist who expects to be obeyed simply because he is a doctor and considers himself an expert at most things in his department. Or again, by the chief technician who insists that his staff arrive on time and then proceeds to arrive half an hour late and take an extended lunch hour himself.

It is apparent to anyone in contact with the top team of pathologist and technician that often there exists, between them, little trust but considerable friction and antipathy. It is uncommon to find a team who agree on the purpose of their department and in which pathologist and chief technician act as a team rather than as two individuals virtually competing against each other for recognition, power and autonomy. This can be so bad that they will communicate only by letter when their offices are adjacent. Even those pathologists who talk about team-work in their own department would be shocked to discover how little team spirit exists and how much distrust and suspicion there is.

PURPOSE OF PATHOLOGY DEPARTMENTS

Before attempting to discuss what sort of organization should be set up and how it should be managed, it is necessary to analyse the work of a pathology department. In the simplest terms, a clinician sends in a specimen, or patient, and a request form on which he has written the name of a test or estimation and receives in return, in the form of a written report, information which is either a measurement, an observation or an opinion. Reports are frequently described as being diagnostic information, but there is considerable doubt about this as a survey has shown that only 3 per cent of biochemistry reports were diagnostic information in that the clinician based his diagnosis on this single piece of information (Bold and Corrin, 1965).

When deciding how well a department is achieving its purpose of providing information, criteria have to be described and since the service is for clinicians their view on what constitutes a good service is the most important. Thus a report must tell a clinician what he wanted to know, the information must be what he has asked for though it may have been obtained by doing a different test from that requested. For example a request may be for bleeding and clotting time but technicians could carry out a screening test for coagulation defects. Again, having been asked for liver function tests, laboratory staff may report a group of tests that they consider are a reasonable screen for liver function but it must be realized that the clinician will only be satisfied if he receives the information he wanted.

Again a report is of no use until it has been seen at the right place, at the right time, by the clinician concerned. So often laboratory staff appear uninterested in the fate of reports once they have been dispatched from the laboratory. The report must arrive in time to be useful and to avoid delaying clinicians in their work but this statement must be qualified and the time of arrival of reports must be considered in conjunction with clinicians' activities. While a report on an out-patient will not be required until the next clinic, or the report on a biopsy may not be required for two or three days when the surgeon does his round, a clinician may need information about a patient's electrolytes or haemoglobin level within an hour. Timing will also be related to the programme followed by clinicians on wards, in theatres or in out-patient clinics. A consultant physician may review his cases every day or every third day, a surgeon may operate every other day or once a week and again a general practitioner may not see his antenatal patient for another month. The arrival of reports must fit in with these programmes, and the assumption that these programmes will be speeded up if pathology reports arrive more quickly is false and no argument in support of a request for extra money or equipment as many seem to think.

A report or information must be presented in such a way that it is easily understood. Clinicians need to have information about the units in which tests are reported, the normal ranges of chemical and cellular constituents and the meaning and significance of standard phrases used in reports involving opinion such as bone marrow or cytology smears. The significance of information should be clearly understood—for example, the accuracy of estimation should be related to differences which have clinical significance. Again a haemoglobin level which shows the first decimal place is misleading for the variation in a patient during the day is more than this indicates. Estimation of substances which have a diurnal variation must be reported with the time of collection of the specimen if a comparison is to be made with results obtained on previous days. Finally reports must be on a form that can easily be stored or filed in a patient's case-notes with the minimum of effort and readily retrieved for reference.

This then is the purpose of a pathology department and these are the criteria for an effective service providing information which may be either a measurement observation or an opinion for clinicians. This purpose can be effectively achieved if reports are received by the clinician: (a) in time to be useful; (b) set out in such a way that the information is easily understood; and (c) on a form that can be easily filed and retrieved.

While it is easy to believe that the only function of a pathology department is to provide information, it must always be remembered that in addition all levels of staff have to be trained and research undertaken not only into clinical problems but also into technology and the organization of work and the department itself. It is both dangerous and short-sighted to lose sight of these other functions for if they are ignored the whole future of the department is jeopardized. Once a student technician, basic grade biochemist or houseman is employed the commitment to train is automatically accepted. If the balance between these three purposes is not kept the department will become inefficient. Staff must learn to measure the amount of effort being spent on each purpose and the use being made of available resources.

Activities Necessary to Achieve Purpose

To achieve these three purposes a number of other activities must be undertaken both inside and outside the department. It is necessary to find out what sort of service clinicians need from the department and in return to explain to them what the department is capable of providing. Future needs must be estimated and used as a basis for asking for money from the H.M.C. Any changes in the hospital programme—such as new out-patient clinics or increases in beds—should be known well in advance, so that the likely demand can be calculated and steps taken to provide the required service. These various activities are carried out within a policy framework, set by the Ministry of Health, Regional Boards and H.M.C. and a department will need to be aware of these policies if it is to work successfully. Professional bodies also create regulations which affect the working situation inside departments. Conditions of service for technicians and biochemists are set by the Whitley Council and for consultants by the Ministry of Health. Information regarding policy and regulations and conditions of service must be collected by a department before it can function satisfactorily.

Within a department, staff, money and work have to be allocated between the various laboratories. Checks have to be made that laboratories are working satisfactorily and statistical information has to be fed back to H.M.C. to confirm that resources are being used economically. The work itself has to be organized and the staff supervised in each laboratory in their daily duties.

TABLE 7
Group of Activities within Pathology Departments

Purpose	Activities	Job
To provide information for clinicians	Assess clinicians needs Obtain money from H.M.C.	Director
Train staff	Change money into resources Allocate resources and work Measure performance	Manager
Research and development	Carry out technical work Train staff Research and development	Technologist

Three main groups of activities can be discerned in this list (*see* Table 7), which departments must undertake, each requiring different approaches and skills. This in turn suggests an organizational structure such as that shown in *Figure 3*. The first group

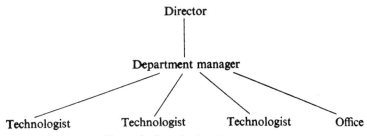

Figure 3. *Organizational structure.*

shown can be described as the director's job; this is to find out how much and what sort of information clinicians require in the future and, with the knowledge of the capability of his department, to claim an annual allocation of money from his H.M.C. in competition with other hospital departments. He can then set out the broad outlines of the range and quality of work, training and research to be undertaken by his department with the available resources.

The second can be described as the departmental manager's job, using money from the H.M.C. for staff equipment and supplies, allocating these and work to the various laboratories within his department and supervising standards of performance. It includes also the collection of statistical information about performance which is to be transmitted to the H.M.C. and also forms the basis for planning future requirements. Service for the pathology department provided by the hospital and external bodies such as technical colleges must be co-ordinated too.

The last job listed in Table 7 is that of the technologist and entails the organization of a laboratory, supervision of staff, training, research and any other activities that take place within the laboratory.

The rank or grade of the person undertaking any of these three jobs must vary with the size of the department. In a small department a chief technician, in the absence of a pathologist, may act as the director while in a very large department it is commonly found that the senior pathologist will do the job of director and other pathologists will act as technologists, as well as consultants. A large biochemistry laboratory will have a biochemist—who may be medically qualified—as technologist but in a smaller one it might be a chief or senior technician. Their performance will then depend on their education and training and their own perception of the job and which part of it they see as important. Whatever grade of person does the job, much of the managerial and supervisory work will be ignored or not done consciously but the grade of that person is of less consequence than whether or not he understands what he is trying to do. All three jobs are invariably done in conjunction with other work such as technology or routine work or—in the case of the pathologist—medical consultation. These latter activities are invariably considered more important and are given priority.

DIRECTOR

This new description and analysis of the activities of a pathology department make it possible to consider how a department can be managed. The director has to assess the needs of hospital clinicians, general practitioners and medical officers of health and the priority of these needs. He also has to be aware of the new developments in medicine—and to a lesser extent in technology—what future activities are being planned for the hospitals and what changes are being considered in the function of the G.P. and M.O.H.

With a knowledge of the capability of his department the director then has to claim money from the H.M.C. in competition with all other hospital departments and he should consider his claim in relation to the needs of the hospital as a whole and the total money available. His claim must be backed by reliable information about future work-load, future hospital activity and statistical information about the work being done with existing staff, space and equipment. It is possible for directors to hoodwink administrators with graphs and statistics but only in the short run and these manoeuvres lead to bad feeling and loss of confidence between administrators and director.

Once the H.M.C. have allocated money for the department, the director must set out in broad terms for the manager, what sort of service should be organized, and what standard of performance he expects; he should also say how much training and research should be undertaken. The director then has to inform clinicians who use the service of what they can expect, the limitations of the service and how best to use it. Although clinicians' needs have priority the director must advise them of what service or information they themselves need and this is not always what they ask for. He has to strike a balance between rigidity of service with the tendency to ignore the needs of clinicians in favour of departmental regulations and total subservience to clinicians and making no use at all in consequence of his own professional expertise. Pathology departments being subject to financial constraint and various regulations are not able to provide an unlimited service. Once clinicians' needs are understood and agreed upon, the director must describe what sort of service will be provided. He will have to set the balance between providing a service, training and research. No one else can do this, clinicians or administrator, as they lack the necessary expertise.

The director will be evading his responsibilities if he implies to clinicians that he is unable to provide a better service because the finance office is not prepared to give him any more money. Rather, he should say that, as the director, he is satisfied that he put in the best possible claim for money and has received an allocation in reasonable proportion to that of other departments and he is organizing his department in what he considers to be the most effective and efficient manner.

Directors' Problems

The job of the director, creates a number of problems for the pathologist. A director is considered to be much the same as an administrator and therefore of a low status in medical circles; consequently the pathologist tends to play down his job as director. He has never received any training for this work and his medical training is a disadvantage in some ways, producing strong individualists rather than team leaders or directors. When a pathologist is promoted to senior consultant he tends to continue to behave as he has always done instead of recognizing the job as an entirely different one. This can have a serious effect as his department is dependent so much on his skill as a director in obtaining a fair allocation of money from the H.M.C. A consultant pathologist, as a professional, has to provide a service for clients who are themselves consultant clinicians, holding equal rank and status, instead of being outside the profession as most clients are (for example, a lawyer and his client or a doctor and his patient). This increases his difficulties when, because of the shortage of money, he may have to limit the service he gives to consultants with whom he seeks equal status and who firmly believe in clinical freedom which they frequently interpret in terms of being entitled to unlimited services. Again in endeavouring to educate clinicians to make the best use of the department the pathologist may appear indirectly to be questioning the efficiency of the clinical team of consultant, registrar and houseman, who are also his colleagues.

The second group of problems facing the pathologist as director is that he has to deal with administrators who are becoming more skilled in making the hospital work as a bureaucratic system. These administrators have authority but when challenged can always, in the final resort, say that the responsibility rests with the Hospital Management Committee. Finally these administrators are now able to look behind the smoke screen which so often hides a pathology department's performance and by using new techniques (*see* Hospital Services O & M Report No. 10, 1967) can measure how efficiently resources are being used in the department. Pathologists have problems about money which arise from the way the total hospital budget is managed as some treasurers seem to be more preoccupied with balancing their books each year than with using money in a positive way to provide a better service.

Finally the pathologist as director faces the problem of being overwhelmed by routine work. He feels that he is becoming subservient to the clinicians yet has great difficulty in delegating responsibility for the work to his staff feeling that he will lose control and eventually become superfluous. He employs qualified biochemists and qualified technicians, yet seems unable to delegate authority and retain responsibility. The A.C.P. further complicate matters by insisting that consultant pathologists are responsible for every activity in their departments.

MANAGER

Discussions between the director and the departmental manager will establish the service to be organized and they will decide upon the range of work to be done and who may send in requests for such work and also upon the broad standards of performance such as unit costs, technicians–request ratio and the general quality of the service: for example, the time taken for a report to reach a clinician. If the manager is allowed to organize the technical service without such standards being agreed upon first, seeds for future disagreement may well be sown. The director and manager must also agree on time to be spent on training and the limits within which technologists can undertake research at their own discretion.

Allocation of Work and Resources

The departmental manager must now ensure that the work is divided into logical groups and the staff organized into teams to carry it out. In most cases, this division of work has been long established by tradition into the four major groups, Haematology, Bacteriology, Biochemistry and Histology, but it is now necessary to reconsider this grouping as new ideas and techniques are developed. In order to allocate staff, money and space accurately, the manager will have to consider past records of performance and have forecasts of future work-loads. Records and forecasts are not infallible but they do reduce the possibility of gross errors.

Setting Objectives

Discussion should now take place betwen manager and technologists on the three main purposes or objectives of each laboratory—that is, routine work, training and research. There should be a clear understanding from the beginning that the manager is concerned with what will be done and not how it will be done, this latter being the concern of the technologist. With regard to routine work the range of tests should be agreed together with standards of performance such as the time taken to produce reports, technician–request ratio, utilization of technicians' time, expenditure on equipment and reagents and utilization of space. The manager must define the amount of training to be done and the progress various grades of staff should be expected to make. In brief the relationship between director, manager and technologist is such that the director describes clinicians' requirements, the manager provides the resources and the technologist provides the techniques.

Setting Standards

The manager has also to set standards of safety to be followed in each laboratory concerning such things as toxic chemicals, electrical equipment and inflammable solvents. Standards must also be set in disciplinary matters such as time-keeping. Technical discipline is generally well understood in relation to producing accurate reports but it is not so clearly understood in relation to safety in general. The manager must set such standards, in delegating authority to technologists, for if a technician is involved in an accident while following the standards laid down then the manager is responsible. If, on the other hand, the technician concerned was not keeping the standards of safety then he is responsible for the accident. If the manager sets standards and takes no action when these standards are not maintained then he is condoning and in effect agreeing to the lower standards.

The three previous paragraphs cover the delegation by the manager of the job of organizing the routine work and training to each technologist together with standards of performance required. The relationship between director, manager and technologist is obviously a triangular one. The director in describing his assessment of clinicians' needs, lays out the broad pattern of technologists' technical work. The manager provides resources and standards of efficiency and effectiveness. The technologist will have to maintain a balance between the three main purposes of his laboratory. Clinicians will complain if the routine work is not done, students will complain and possibly leave if their training is inadequate and, without research, laboratory staff will tend to lose their sparkle and enthusiasm. The way in which these objectives are set and standards agreed are probably the key to the way in which managers continue to train and educate technologists and help or impede, as the case may be, in their development as people and as future departmental managers. Information must be supplied to the technologist to enable him to keep a check on the efficiency of his laboratory for he needs to know how many requests arrive each month, how much money he is spending, the ratio of staff to requests, and the sickness and absentee rate among his staff. If any of these figures indicate that something is wrong the technologist can then take immediate action to find the cause and remedy the situation if possible. It is of no value to compare the number of requests received by different laboratories in a department as so often it can lead to intergroup competition and its attendant problems (Schein, 1965). What must be decided is whether each laboratory's performance is improving from year to year and if investment in automated equipment, for example, is being reflected in more requests being processed by the same number of staff.

It is a debatable point whether the office in a pathology department should be considered as an integral part of the department or as a service to the department. But the manager must discuss and get agreement with the senior clerical assistant regarding the purpose of the office and standards of performance. There must be a clear understanding between them that the purpose of the office is: firstly to receive requests and specimens, to record the type of work and the source, dispatch reports to clinicians and file a copy; secondly provision of a clerical service for the director, manager and technologists (in the case of technologists, some resentment may be met but it is essential that they are relieved of unnecessary clerical work); thirdly to undertake the clerical work involved in the ordering of supplies and control of stores; and finally, to maintain staff records. Standards of performance can then be agreed between the manager, senior clerical assistant and the hospital records officer for each of these purposes, together with a programme for sending out reports.

Ordering Supplies and Equipment

Ordering stores and controlling stocks are considered to be dull but necessary chores but this can be useful in that it gives the manager an easy method of supervising and controlling all activities in the department especially if he has not sufficient authority to supervise in any better way. It is only necessary to consider how much money is tied up in stores, the cost of maintaining the space it occupies, the disastrous effect when one item runs out and work is held up, the cost of placing an order, checking receipt, certifying invoice for payment and issuing stores to laboratories to appreciate how much time is spent on this job. Information on techniques for simplifying this work is available and Oxford Regional Board O & M Department have investigated ways of calculating the most economical amounts to order and the ideal frequency of ordering to avoid running out. Stock level indicators, bin cards, records of supplier and costs with lead times will all make the work simpler. Annual contracts and the use of existing regional bulk contracts will save repetitive ordering. It is important that the manager should always delegate purely clerical work, when possible, to his clerical staff. Experience shows that they are more than capable of doing this work.

The task of issuing stores and writing requisitions is time consuming and has little to recommend it. Signed requisitions are an uncertain method of controlling consumption or avoiding waste as many who sign them will have realized. There is much to be said for topping-up systems. In this system a stock level is agreed upon—the actual level being regulated to useage and storage space. Each week the stocks are made up by a porter to the agreed level from the main stores. The stock level may be an agreed number or shelf space or height (if boxes on a shelf). Take as an example microscope slides; the agreed stock level for haematology may be twelve boxes and for histology seven. Each week the porter will call and make good the slides that have been used in the respective laboratory. This avoids requisitions, issuing by senior staff and reduces the chance of running out of stock.

Recruiting Staff

The manager has to provide technologists with staff, who can either be recruited as qualified staff or as students to be trained in the post. He should supervise this training process by keeping in close touch with the local technical college which provides the necessary courses. Technical Colleges provide a service for pathology departments and it is essential to see both that they are supplying what is required and that the two activities, training and education, match up together; the only person to do this is the department manager. A strong case can be made for including in general studies an understanding of the health service, of the organization of a hospital and of the behaviour of groups of people at work. This gives students encouragement to explore their immediate experience and to understand the organization in which they work and its purpose. Managers should consider the short-term training needs of qualified technicians and ask their local technical colleges to provide short courses on such subjects as molecular biology, microphotography, cytology and immunology, which have come into prominence since many technicians qualified. The same applies to non-technical subjects such as organization of work and supervision; there is at present, only one technical college in the country that offers such a course.

Managers should consider the value of short courses organized by the Institute for it is difficult to see what effect such courses have on the routine work. A manager who draws up a list of short courses attended by his staff over the last two years will see that little information came into his department as a result. These courses are good for morale and are an opportunity for meeting other technicians but this is not their primary purpose. Part of the failure lies with the organizers in designing a course in which some 200 experienced technicians listen to someone delivering a lecture which they could just as well have read. Questions after this sort of lecture are rarely illuminating. Some alternative form must be developed which will actively involve the participants practically and intellectually. Managers on their part could insist that staff attending these courses should provide a written report for the benefit of other members of the staff and as a record of the lectures or work.

When a technician has acquired special skill and experience as a result of attending a course or been given an opportunity to develop these during working hours an effort should be made by the manager to see that they are rapidly passed on to other members of the staff. This will avoid the considerable loss of expertise that can occur when this technician leaves the department for another post.

The manager should organize the flow of information into his department. Scientific, medical and trade journals should be circulated—each technologist indicating that he has seen them. He should also know how to obtain reprints for staff from the less well known or more specialized journals. Textbooks are a more difficult problem, for technologists need one range and students will need a different one; all of these have to be paid for.

One member of the technical staff should be made responsible for receiving all the technical journals that come into the department and ensuring that they are circulated to each individual laboratory. A simple system of signing the appropriate form can be used to check that every laboratory has seen the journal and the responsible person would then file the latter. In each laboratory one person could be responsible for reviewing one or more journals and bringing relevant articles to the attention of some or all of the technical staff. Arrangements should be made for relevant technical information to be filed in each department. It should be made quite clear that this information belongs to the laboratory and not to the individual technician, to avoid the senior technician taking it with him when he leaves for another job. Photocopying a useful article is a better method than tearing journals apart and a modest expenditure of £100 on photocopying will be money well spent in helping to provide each laboratory with readily accessible information. Circulation of a technical journal is no guarantee that it will be read; indeed there is evidence to suggest that technicians in general read very few of them. Finally, the most sought after information—in the Whitley Council's P.T.B. Circulars on salaries and conditions of service and relevant H.M. circulars—has the most limited circulation for reasons it is difficult to understand.

CO-ORDINATING SERVICE PROVIDED BY THE HOSPITAL

The hospital secretary provides a number of services such as engineering, building maintenance, portering and cleaning, all of which must be co-ordinated within the pathology department by the manager. A technologist should understand the conditions under which he may make use of them, for though they are essential to the efficient running of the department they cost money so must be used economically. The hospital secretary provides other services such as recruiting staff and transmitting policy from H.M.C., Regional Board and Ministry of Health. He also acts as a link with the Group Secretary, Supplies Officer and Treasurer. It makes interdepartmental relationships smoother if the manager knows the heads of the various departments providing these services, if not personally, at least by name and where they can be found. He should also know something of the organization of the services.

Co-ordination of Laboratories

There is a range of activities that has to be organized by the departmental manager and co-ordinated with the activities of the department. For example a technologist must co-operate by sending out reports to the office in good time for processing and dispatching; domestic staff must clean laboratories without interfering with the work; laboratories sharing equipment must work together. Co-ordinating the complex activities of pathology departments calls for an effective departmental manager. There is no single way of doing this job as it depends on many things such as the character of the director, the way the department is organized and relationships between staff. The manager has a personal responsibility for seeing that technicians co-operate in getting the work done and training staff. He cannot afford the luxury of opting out of difficult situations or defending his position or principles without the whole department suffering or becoming less efficient as a result of strained relationships between manager and technologist or manager and director.

The usual activity within pathology departments can be represented diagrammatically as follows.

Receipt of ⟶ Estimation ⟶ Recording ⟶ Reporting
specimen   results

However this is only part of the whole process which is more accurately described in the following way.

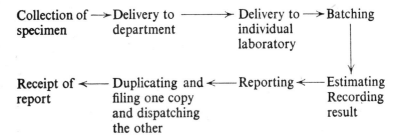

There is need for an overall view of this complex system to avoid changes being made in one section which will throw the other out of gear. Each part of the system must be related to the other parts. Advantages derived from changes from manual to automated methods may be neutralized by the inability of office staffs to cope with the extra reports. A laboratory programme which delivers reports to the office a few minutes before it closes is not efficient. The manager has a great co-ordinating role to play in this area and should be familiar with the system as a whole and have details of programmes in wards, theatres and Out-patient departments as well as his own office and laboratories.

The introduction of automated equipment means that the manager has to attempt to control the input of work into the various laboratories. This can be facilitated by technical staff collecting all the blood samples from in-patients first thing in the morning and a porter collecting all other specimens from wards and delivering them to the laboratories. In this way the technologist can safely predict when 90 per cent of his work will arrive and plan his day accordingly. Any change in clinical programmes such as a new out-patient clinic or new day for theatre work can be assessed and fitted in to the existing laboratory programme. This is a better alternative than 30 diabetic patients arriving out of the blue requiring blood sugar estimations. As the pressures on hospitals grow the departmental manager will have to watch the clinical programme more closely and be able to adjust his laboratory programme to meet alterations in demand for work.

One method of simplifying and improving co-ordination is to hold regular meetings of senior staff to discuss matters relating to more than one laboratory in the department—such as the collection of specimens mentioned on page 66. Meeting of staff engaged on a common task such as 'on-call' can iron out problems quickly and efficiently and go a long way to avoiding misunderstandings arising. These meetings give the senior staff an opportunity to express their views and to hear what other senior staff think. While this method of co-ordinating has much to recommend it, some chief technicians will find themselves subject to considerable pressure from senior staff and may be forced to use other methods for co-ordinating activities.

Finally the departmental manager has to measure the work done by the department in terms of efficiency and effectiveness. Statistics provided by the office staff, should clearly indicate how much work has been done in the previous month and the number of staff who have been absent for any reason. It can then be calculated how effectively technical staff are being used and the figures passed back both to the technologist so that he is aware of the performance of his staff, and to the medical records officer who builds them into the record of the performance of the hospital as a whole. This record (SBH 6) is sent to the Regional Board who calculate unit costs for all departments, enabling managers to compare current performance with previous performance. The figures can also be used by the H.M.C. as a rough guide to how well the pathology department is using its resources and also by the departmental manager to forecast future work-loads and future requirements of staff, money and equipment.

It is much more difficult for the manager to check on the effectiveness of the department in providing a service that is meeting clinicians' requirements. He needs to have open and undistorted lines of communication with them and to be able to check informally and on a personal basis. Housemen change jobs every six months and it is therefore difficult to reach any understanding with them, but a registrar stays longer and is probably the best person to approach. General practitioners occasionally call in at the department and an attempt should be made to find out from them if they are satisfied with the service generally.

MANAGEMENT PROBLEMS

In practice there are serious problems for the chief technician who sees himself as a departmental manager. He has not had specialized training for such activities as planning or managing technologists and so has to learn by experience, always a slow, painful and uncertain process. His job has probably never been described to him and he has no clear idea how far his authority extends and consequently suffers from indecision. He has, in practice, three part-time jobs as technologist, administrator and manager. As a technologist he runs an individual laboratory within the department. As an administrator he collects and transmits information regarding such matters as work-loads and receipt of goods and also authorizes actions taken within a clearly defined set of rules such as arranging holidays, issuing stores and works orders. As manager he will be involved in planning, converting resources and allocating work and resources. Generally chief technicians write their own job description and in consequence some underestimate and others overestimate the job. Pathologists rarely define precisely either how much authority and responsibility should be delegated to the technologist by the chief technician or the relationship between biochemist and chief technician. On promotion he tends, in consequence, to go on behaving like a good technologist instead of carrying out the new job as departmental manager.

The pathologist's attitude also creates problems for his departmental manager since he invariably experiences great difficulty in delegating duties without losing control of the work. He is apprehensive of not knowing everything that is going on in the department so he hesitates to lay down any sort of policy; this means all decisions have to come back to him to be settled. Pathologists as a rule, have no clear understanding of the function of their chief technician and will frequently take over his job whenever they feel like it, so undermining his authority.

Problems are also created for the chief technician as manager by technologists for they tend to look down on administrative staff in general and administrative chief technicians in particular and do not understand his essential managerial function in the department—that of planning, allocating and co-ordinating.

Many a chief technician will experience a conflict of loyalties between his profession and his responsibilities as departmental manager. Decisions about the widespread use of unqualified staff such as laboratory aides who are good for the department but bad for the profession are a good example of such a conflict. Chief technicians derive much of their status from being the exclusive holders of particular technical skills. But today it is not so easy for them to be the exclusive holder of technical skills, partly because of the pressure of work. To compensate for this some chief technicians are making enormous efforts to acquire higher academic qualifications in order to be able to retain their high status. Unfortunately managerial skills, not being one of the professional aspirations of technicians, do not confer high status. As a result few chief technicians make any real effort to become the exclusive holders of managerial skills in spite of the fact that these skills are directly related to the work they do.

Delegation

Although it is not intended to discuss managerial skills to any great extent in this chapter, there are two skills which seem important and yet are misunderstood in pathology departments. The first involves delegation which the Concise Oxford dictionary defines as 'to commit authority to an agent to carry out a task'. Everyone would agree that the task must be clearly described and standards of performance set (for example, time to be taken or cost) if the agent is to carry out the task successfully. The distinction between delegating a task and giving a series of commands can be illustrated in the following way. When an agent has been delegated authority to carry out a task he is responsible for how the task is performed within the limits or standards of performance that have been set. When an agent receives a set of detailed commands he is not responsible for how the overall task is achieved as he is simply carrying out the commands.

A pathologist, responsible for providing a pathology service, does not lose authority or control when he delegates the job of organizing a laboratory to a technician or biochemist. He fulfils his responsibility by delegating a job to a person who is satisfactorily qualified and experienced and capable of doing the job in question. The pathologist is still responsible for ensuring the service is provided but the technician is responsible for the job and should have the authority to decide how he does it. Delegation makes little sense if it simply means that somebody has to undertake part of the delegator's work. It is not true to say that he is the best sort of manager who has delegated all his work. However at present many people doing the job of director or manager in

69

pathology departments are doing an enormous amount of work which does not require their skill or experience and could easily be done by others, leaving the director or manager with more time to get the more important things done.

Delegation must be done skilfully for it is not sufficient to say to a new technologist: 'you are to run the haematology laboratory; we do not worry much about rules and regulations here and I give technologists a free hand in running their laboratories'. The technologist will feel pleased with his new manager or director for giving him a free hand. A few weeks later the manager may well have to ask the technologist why he threw out a certain technique, or why he kept a consultant surgeon waiting for two hours before sending him a haemoglobin result, commenting: 'you should have known better and asked me first'. The technologist is unlikely to remind him about being given a free hand and will accept the rebuke. Slowly over the next few years the technologist will learn all the unwritten rules concerning his laboratory, but each new technologist who takes over this haematology laboratory will have to go through the same slow and uncertain learning process. Delegation could be more satisfactory if the rules were thought about and described, as far as possible, to each new technologist and better still if they were written down. A technologist may object to this apparently detailed delegation but in fact it gives him a far greater freedom of action for he knows how far his authority extends and the standards of performance. Chief technicians who pride themselves on a liberal or non-restrictive approach are unable to see that such an approach increases problems of this kind. The whole subject of delegating responsibility and authority has been widely explored by Brown (1960).

Communicating

The other important managerial skill is in communicating. Pathology departments are under considerable pressure to meet the changing needs of clinicians, they are subject to innumerable emergencies and success under these conditions will only be assured if there is a free flow of information within the department. Analysis of the day-to-day activities of a departmental manager shows that he spends much of his time in communicating with the technologist and to a smaller extent with his director and other hospital departments. It is essential that all three groups improve their skill in communications and appreciate the influences that make communication more or less intelligible. A further discussion on

70

the wider implications of communications will be included in Chapter 6.

SUMMARY

An attempt has been made in this chapter to analyse the purpose of pathology departments, discuss activities that are necessary to achieve this purpose and describe the various jobs that emerge from the discussion. Each arrow in *Figure 4* indicates a flow of resources or services into the department and, equally important, an outward flow of accurate information.

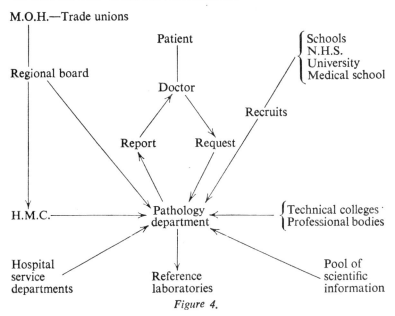

Figure 4.

In practice these jobs are not clear-cut activities but are carried out at the same time as the medical or scientific work; thus the pathologist will also have his work as a consultant and the chief technician may have to do a technologist's job as well. Both will be involved in innumerable minor problems. Directing and managing a department are not obvious activities nor are they easily carried out; they tend to get pushed to one side because of the great load of other pressing work and problems. It is most important that directors and managers should allow time for these particular functions, which probably have more effect on the efficiency and effectiveness of the department than anything else.

CHAPTER 4

LABORATORY SUPERVISION AND THE TECHNOLOGIST

INTRODUCTION

For the purpose of this chapter and as described in the previous one, a technologist is a qualified person in charge of a laboratory in a pathology department with responsiblity for running it, organizing the work and supervising the staff. He will have knowledge of the analytical principles used and have authority to make decisions on the methods used and the range of work. This job may be carried out by a pathologist, biochemist or technician depending on circumstances and on the particular size of the laboratory. How he does the job will depend on his training and perception of the job. A pathologist, for example, will tend to delegate much of the technologist's job to the senior person in his laboratory and will be more interested in the diagnostic aspects of the work. A biochemist will delegate less of this work but will be more interested in biochemical problems than in diagnosis. A technician will delegate very little and will be most interested in getting the work done and providing a service.

In spite of these differences a technologist has three main parts to his job, apart from the scientific one—although this may be the most important in his eyes. He must organize the routine work and so provide a service for clinicians; train various grades of staff—and this includes technical and non-technical training; and, finally, undertake research in the broadest sense whether it be in medicine, technology or simply new methods. The technologist has to learn to keep a balance between these three components and this means measuring them and allocating time and resources to each in an order of priority to be decided upon between technologist, departmental manager and director.

In the previous chapter it was pointed out that the technologist, departmental manager and director would discuss and agree on the service to be provided, the amount of training and resources to be allocated to research and also agree the standards of performance, such as staff request ratios and total expenditure. This triangular relationship will be considerably modified by the qualification of the person filling the technologists job.

Measuring Work-load

Once these discussions have been completed, the technologist has to organize his resources of staff, equipment and space to get the work done efficiently. There is no single way of doing this as laboratories vary so much and it is only possible to describe the organizing process itself. First of all, such information will be needed as the amount of work, the variation of the work-load from day to day and the peak times for delivery of specimens which will be related to the activities of clinicians and the arrangements for bringing specimens to the department. The technologist will also need to know the programme organized by the department's office for processing and sending out reports to avoid unnecessary effort to finish work not required for several days. Information will also be needed about the range of tests and the frequency of each test so that decisions can be made regarding whether to use flow or batch methods.

Organizing

Having obtained all possible information, the technologist is now in a position so to deploy his staff as to make the best use of them while providing them with satisfying jobs. Tests can be arranged in groups and be allocated to a small team of technicians, relating the size and range of skill of the team to the probable amount and range of work to be done. As the work-load varies by up to 50 per cent from day to day, there is a tendency to staff for peak work-loads and to ignore what happens during the troughs.

Attention should be paid to simplification of work by mechanical aids and, where the work-load is large enough, to full mechanization. To avoid the technicians becoming bored—a symptom of an unsatisfying job—efforts should be made to enlarge their jobs and make them responsible for either a wider section or taking specimens through to the reporting stage when this is practical. Job simplification without job enlargement will soon produce dissatisfied and bored technicians. A recent report (Hospital Services O & M Report No. 10, 1967) shows that technicians may spend less than 50 per cent of their time doing technical work and that with good organization on the part of the technologist this figure can be increased to 60 per cent. Technicians cannot be expected to be enthusiastic about carrying out one group of tests for ever and should be rotated often enough to maintain enthusiasm and yet not interfere with standards of performance.

The technologist will have to plan the distribution of equipment even though this is invariably restricted by the physical layout of the building. Time can be saved and life made easier for technicians by the optimum placing of equipment in relation to them, the type of work to be done and the frequency with which it is used. There are a number of simple techniques evolved from Work Study which can be used, such as flow diagrams and multiple activity charts, which readily provide information relating to optimum siting of equipment and reagents. Technicians are the most expensive ingredient in a laboratory and the work should be grouped around the team for this saves unnecessary movement and is more satisfying to the team as a whole. In some cases it may be cheaper to buy another centrifuge for example than to have technicians walking into another room to use one. There may be some restriction on the siting of some equipment because of its nature or because it gives off certain dangerous fumes. These considerations only relate to existing laboratories and are not intended for planning new laboratories which would require a comprehensive study.

Information of various types is rarely deliberately and systematically collected although it is essential to the laboratory. Medical, scientific and trade journals should be reviewed and useful information filed for future reference. Information on the performance of the laboratory must be collected—such as accuracy of estimations and test request ratios—but with the minimum of effort. The technologist will need to assess the performance of automated equipment, how often it breaks down, cost of maintenance and when a replacement will be required.

Finally the technologist should try to organize that most valuable commodity—his own time. To discover how he actually spends his time a technologist should occasionally keep a diary of all activities for a week, take a good hard look at it to see what he actually does and then ask himself if he could arrange his programme to greater advantage.

Implementation

Once the technologist has settled the grouping of technicians and the allocation of work he will give a series of orders for the work to be carried out. Staff are more likely to carry out orders willingly if they understand their reason and purpose. One of the great changes which has taken place outside pathology departments since senior staff were at school is that children are now taught in a more permissive way and are more likely to question orders than to obey them implicitly as would have happened 20 years ago. In the same way as the technologist will appreciate the director or manager discussing changes in the department with him so technicians are more likely to follow orders if the technologist discusses them rather than simply issues them. All staff need to understand both the orders and the purpose of the laboratory.

The technologist and his senior technicians should agree on how much work each member or group of staff is capable of with the available equipment. It is a dangerous fallacy to assume that technicians can work at a rapid pace all day or at a pace equal to that which the technologist can maintain for half an hour or so. On the other hand technicians must understand the importance of keeping to a timetable and appreciate the complexity of the organization of the department's office and the circumstances which determine their timetable.

It is well worth while for technologists to plan the regular maintenance of equipment particularly the more complex sort as this greatly reduces the chances of breakdown and its consequent problems. When ordering equipment some advantage can be gained from standardization, where practical, for this reduces the number of spares kept in stock and allows equipment to be transferred temporarily to avoid delays due to breakdown or servicing.

There is much to be said for the use of written standard methods as they help to ensure a level standard of performance, reducing the limits of variations in accuracy. It saves technicians from having to consult a textbook when they undertake a particular test for the first few times and reduces the disruption that can be caused by an experienced technician being away sick or leaving at short notice. Past experience in the laboratory suggests that standard methods are in effect the simplest and most effective way that has been found to carry out tests and provide a method of transferring some of the skill and experience from one technician to the next. They should include the source of the method, reagents, procedure, calculation, faults if any, life of reagents and range of normal values. They have an authority of their own and staff are more likely to follow them if they are in any doubt. It is far better for a technician to read instructions than call across the laboratory to another technician for guidance.

Measuring Performance

The technologist having delegated work to his technicians now has to measure their performance or better still to get them to measure

75

their performance to see if they are achieving their objectives, maintaining the required standards of accuracy, and if each group is doing a reasonable amount of work. Some records have to be kept for this purpose but compiling records is time-consuming and expensive and so they should be kept to a minimum. Having decided what information he needs the technologist should then design the simplest possible system that can provide it. On no account should these records ever be used to criticize the level of performance of the staff. The technologist should also check approximately 10 per cent of the reports leaving the department's office one day a week, to see that reports are legible and leaving the office in good time. The office should provide him with the number of requests received by his laboratory each month and the technologist has to record the number of tests and requests on 12 days during the year.

It is the responsibility of the technologist to see that his staff are reaching the accepted level of efficiency. These records will enable him to discuss with the departmental manager, on a basis of fact, next year's requirements. The technologist will also know what is going on in his laboratory and be able to correct faults soon after they have been observed. Again, he will know the work-load and how it relates to the total number of staff and therefore have facts to put before the departmental manager when asking for extra staff. This avoids the emotional appeal for more staff or money so often made by the technologist who feels his laboratory is overworked but is unable to prove it. Any queries from the departmental manager regarding problems can be answered factually.

Quality Control

The traditional method of using quality control is to take an unknown sample in each batch of sera being tested. The results are accepted only if the result of the unknown sample falls within a narrow range around its true value. If the result is outside the range the technician will have to repeat the batch of tests. As the technologist assumes his staff are not trustworthy they tend to adjust the results of so-called unknown sera to avoid repeating the batch. The real value of quality control is when it is given to the technician doing the tests, its use explained, and he is able freely to accept or reject the batch himself and to identify and correct causes of variation. In other words to encourage personnel to be honest and to investigate variations in estimations. The integrity of technicians is much the same as that of biochemists and pathologists. Quality control can also distinguish between well-trained and poorly-trained technicians and between technicians overstressed and those free from stress. The remedies for both these faults are in the hands of the technologist. The recent introduction of new methods, cumulative summation of results and distribution of results about the normal are helping technologists to achieve a better understanding of controls.

TRAINING

Training is not a popular activity with anyone in pathology departments and many will avoid doing it if they can by insisting that work is piling up. Training has the lowest priority although the future of the department may well depend upon the adequate training of all professional groups. There is some general advice for the technologist who has to train staff which may make life a little easier and the task a little less arduous. The following comments are primarily concerned with training technicians but are equally true for pathologists and biochemists.

To begin with, a timetable should be prepared showing what the student must learn, how much skill he must acquire and what job he should be able to do, how well and how soon. Secondly the technologist must be familiar with the principles involved, preferably having them written down, and knowing which textbook gives a suitable description of these principles. These can be included in the standard methods. Thirdly, the technique must be broken down into essential parts or key points. Finally, everything should be ready before beginning—the equipment and reagents being laid out just as when the technique is being done routinely. If everything is laid out in the correct order the student is more likely to follow the correct pattern. When it comes to the training itself the student should be put at his ease—he won't think properly if he is embarrassed or nervous. It is important to find out what he already knows and start him where his knowledge ends so that he is not bored by repetition. His interest in learning must be aroused and the relationship of his work to the function and work of the laboratory made clear so that he can appreciate its importance. He should next be placed in the correct position with the equipment and reagents laid out as in routine work and the principles explained in sufficient detail for him to understand. The techniques must then be presented to him and the key points, which will make or break it, explained. He should be questioned to see if he has really understood and grasped the technique and it may be necessary to repeat the explanations and to make quite sure that he really understands the principle involved. This will lead to fewer mistakes. His performance should then be tried out by having him carry out the technique while explaining the main points; this is a very useful procedure. It is essential at this stage to be patient with him and to go slowly for it is important to get accuracy first and speed later. The reason for the controls which must be built into the technique should be explained; he must understand that they are indicators for his use and will show him when something has gone wrong, so that he can go back and check what he has done.

Finally when he seems to have the feel of the technique, he must be allowed to do it by himself with someone to supervise him and to whom he can go if he needs help. The job should not be taken away from him too soon or too often if he appears to be going wrong; indeed it should not be taken over at all if it is possible to point out the errors and how he should correct them. This coaching can then be tapered off until he is able to work under routine supervision. It will be found useful with student technicians to make them keep some sort of written record of the technical work they do in the laboratory. This not only shows what progress they are making but also enables the technologist to check the actual work they are doing for comprehension as the extent of this soon shows up in even a brief written description of the technique.

EDUCATION

Training by itself is only half the problem for student technicians; the rest might be described as education and helping them to develop a potential for becoming senior technicians and technologists. This educational and development process must be part of the way in which the technologist handles his staff. Young people need a framework of rules within which to learn how to behave and discipline is best exerted by persuasion rather than enforced by punishment. The strongest discipline is exerted by fellow technicians who make up the informal groups in the laboratory and intelligent supervisors should accept this fact; constant nagging, threats or punishment simply create deep resentment.

When tackling disciplinary problems concerning staff there are a few guide-lines which may be helpful. All the facts about the individual concerned and the problem should be collected and the rules and customs that may affect the problem noted for there are many of these in every department. The appropriate people should be asked for their opinion and feelings about both the problem and the facts surrounding it. These facts can then be fitted together and their relationship one with another considered so that any gaps or contradictions are noted and if necessary more facts obtained. Then it is possible to come to some decision as to what is to be accomplished, taking into consideration what effect it should have on the individual, the rest of the staff and the laboratory. It will then be possible to decide upon the most satisfactory solution both for the person concerned and for the laboratory. The necessary action being taken, changes in attitude, relationships and the effect on the work should be noted for, by solving this particular problem, others may be produced.

In handling a group of people the technologist needs to have some understanding of his own motives and of the very human need for everyone to belong to a group which supports him and to which he can contribute and above all the need to do a meaningful job. He must understand something of the behaviour and strength of informal groups among staff, the defence mechanisms of these groups when attacked, a man's need for status particularly among his own group and his need to be accepted by his boss as a human being with feeling and not treated as an automaton and finally his need to have some control over his own future. A technologist should be aware of these needs in his own staff, in other hospital staff and particularly in himself.

Purpose of Training and Education

In carrying out this training and education what are we trying to achieve? First of all it is hoped to create a successful working group. In the case of the individual technician, as they should above all be technically competent, the bulk of their training is directed in this way but also they must develop the capacity for taking decisions, for keeping their head when things go wrong and the ability to get on with people. So the technologist himself must not only set an example in the way he supervises his staff but he must also give them, individually, the opportunity to practise taking decisions and supervising small groups of technicians; without this they will never become competent. If they are permitted occasionally to decide their own course of action and to understand and accept the consequences of this or if they are allowed to run a small team in their own way they will gain confidence and experience. The technologist may find it difficult to step aside but in the long run he will find it much easier than taking all their decisions for them.

PROBLEMS OF TECHNOLOGISTS

What are the problems facing the various people doing a technologist's job? A pathologist in charge of a laboratory will often be underemployed and need to fill in his time with research or technical work. He will be interested rather in acting as a consultant and in the medical aspects of the work than as a technologist; supervising and organizing it, in consequence, but at the same time only being prepared to delegate a small part of it to his senior technician although the latter probably knows more of technology. His need to maintain his public image with other consultant clinicians will also affect his behaviour to some extent. His experience and training do not include the supervision of a group of technicians or the organization of work and in some ways inhibit successful relationships with technicians.

A biochemist has different problems. When, after graduating, he takes a post as a technologist he has no knowledge of medicine, hospitals or pathology departments or of the people who work in them. His training has been orientated to research and has not included principles of analysis or instrumentation. He does not belong with nor is he likely to be accepted by either group—pathologists or technicians. He has not been trained to organize work and he must adjust to the idea of providing a service.

A technician promoted to the job of technologist tends to go on behaving as a good technician instead of accepting and carrying out the new duties. He will accept more readily the idea of providing a service for clinicians although this will depend to some extent on the particular type of laboratory in which he works as explained previously. He tends to see technology as his personal expertise feeling that from this he derives his status rather than from his supervisory skill. Not every technician has sufficient scientific training to be a technologist for today the qualification of F.I.M.L.T. is insufficient by itself unless it has been backed up with a good deal of studying.

All three groups consider work-organization and work-supervision to have low priority. When a clever technician becomes a technologist he will continue his studies to become a better technologist; by studying for example, for a degree, but never to become a departmental manager. None of the professional bodies give any training in work-organization and work-supervision or first-line management as it is known today. A technologist's shortcomings may not be obvious when in charge of 2 or 3 technicians but they will be painfully so when the number reaches 20.

It is useful to consider how pathologists see the job of a technologist when it is being done by a biochemist or technician. The majority simply expect technologists to get the work done under their direction and technicians to do their technical work conscientiously and quickly and supervise other technicians. Pathologists rarely give more consideration to the job than this. It is unusual to find one explaining or describing the job in detail to a new technologist. A pathologist does not expect a technologist to discuss results with doctors or to understand the meaning of reports nor does he take much interest in the training technologists give to their students. Neither do many pathologists appear to consider it necessary for technologists to understand the theories on which techniques are based, though good results are dependent on this. Although they do identical jobs, technicians and biochemists are treated very differently simply because the latter are graduates. A chief technician may be running a haematology laboratory with 20 technicians but will tend to be treated as inferior to a graduate biochemist with a staff of 3 and a smaller laboratory.

Finally, how do technicians see their technologist? This must depend on the performance of the individual technologist as at one extreme their attitude will be cynical because they know he simply carries out the detailed orders given to him by the pathologist and has very little say of his own. At the other end of the scale when he is progressive, encourages and trains his staff, keeps up to date and provides a thoroughly satisfying job for his students, they will appreciate his efforts and give him loyalty.

It is hard to understand why the technologist is treated so indifferently for he is the key man who gets the work done, checks results, motivates the staff, sees that reagents and equipment are in working order and checks accuracy. He is the person who influences the actual test carried out in the department. One of the difficulties is that the job was never designed—it simply grew out of the job of unskilled personal assistant to pathologists which obtained 50 years ago. The technologist is expected to be an expert technician, an expert supervisor and an expert at organizing work. How he acquires this expertise is left to chance. The job is now obviously becoming complex.

The technologist of today may be a good supervisor in his face-to-face relations with his staff but on promotion to departmental manager he may not be prepared to manage a large department by organizing work and jobs, by planning or in other words through managing resources. Large departments cannot be managed through personal relationships and so once the technologist becomes a departmental manager his methods must become impersonal when he sets objectives, plans and organizes his department. The emphasis for the technologist will always be on direct personal supervision but there should be some opportunity for experience or training in managing departments.

TRAINING TECHNOLOGISTS IN SUPERVISION

For many years the view was that good technologists were born not made but this view is changing and it is now thought that possibly technologists can be trained to supervise. The experience outside pathology departments in the training of supervisors has not been very successful and it is now felt that supervisors can only be trained on the basis of an analysis of the actual job they do. The necessary skills and knowledge can then be established.

For the moment promotion from technician to technologist is governed mainly by qualifications and ability to get the technical work done; skill in supervising staff is not considered. A job analysis will provide the material for developing training courses for future technologists; it will also provide a description which can then be discussed by the technologist and his superiors to make sure they both understand the job. The difficult question concerns who will undertake this analysis, as staff in pathology departments are very busy. One possibility is to ask the Organization and Method Study Department, available in most regions, to assist. But the director and departmental manager must be involved in this analysis if the training is to be of any value because it will inevitably entail reassessment of jobs and clarification, between manager and director, as to what the technologist's job is. It may mean reviewing existing attitudes and organization. Without whole-hearted co-operation between the person carrying out the analysis and the director and manager, the exercise is doomed to failure. This new approach to training of supervisors is described in *Supervisory Training: A New Approach for Management* published by H.M. Stationery Office (1966).

Once this analysis has been done in a number of departments and a general pattern has begun to appear it will be possible to plan a course for technicians before they take up the post of technologist. This need only be a short course but it should prove much more satisfactory than the present system of placing a newly appointed technologist in charge of a group of technicians and just hoping for the best. As this training will cost money, it is essential to check its effectiveness with directors and departmental managers, making sure it is meeting the technologist's needs. Training needs to be continuous as a single-shot system of training rarely succeeds. So far Regional Board Training Departments have provided a few courses but these have been concerned with general techniques used in administration rather than with specific skills required by technologists. At the moment the Ministry of Health is stressing interdisciplinary training and with good reason (Schein, 1965) but what is required is training with a single discipline— pathology—but multiprofessional training to include pathologists, biochemists and technicians.

There are some problems which will not be solved by training and require alterations in the organization of pathology departments. The job of the technologist needs simplification as he is at present responsible for too many things. The introduction of automated equipment means that a larger percentage of his time is spent in handling request and report forms and this could well be done by a clerical assistant. This again, brings up the problem of the relationship between the technologist and the office staff which is often unsatisfactory. The technologist needs a better description of what he is supposed to do, the objectives of his laboratory, how far his authority extends and standards of performance. None of these are laid out clearly enough. If the technologist is to be responsible for the performance of his laboratory then he should have facts about that performance.

SUMMARY

A technologist must be able to organize his laboratory to achieve the objectives of the department and maintain a balance between routine work, training and research. He must be able to forecast the amount and range of work and the staff, reagents and equipment needed to do this work. Furthermore the technologist must be able to create a team out of the staff in his laboratory and be capable of managing and measuring his laboratory's performance He must also train and develop future technicians. He must be willing and able to communicate information to his manager and director and also to his staff. The technologist must be able to motivate his staff and obtain their active support and the interest of his manager and the director. To do this he will have to learn the principles of supervision and work-organization and to see the work in his laboratory in relation not only to the pathology department as a whole but also to the hospital.

CHAPTER 5

MANAGEMENT TECHNIQUES

INTRODUCTION

The previous chapters brought the jobs of director, manager and technologist into sharp focus and some of the techniques used by the manager will now be considered. Personnel management, a type of skill concerning recruitment and training of staff is a large subject and will be covered separately in Chapter 6. Management techniques fall into two main groups: those concerned with planning and organizing resources and controlling performance and those concerned with people, their personality and their behaviour at work. The latter will be described in Chapter 7.

Regional Boards have created Work Study Teams or to use the more common title Organization and Method Study Teams (O & M). These are available on request to all H.M.C.'s and all hospital departments. For many years they have made a valuable contribution to the running efficiency of hospitals and their departments. However it has become evident that the scope of O & M teams is too limited and there is now a tendency to create a more versatile team called Management Services, to provide hospitals and their departments with a wide range of managerial skills such as operational research, manpower planning, systems analysis, forecasting and many other techniques.

Managers can accept management services as a panacea to all their problems hopefully grasping at each new technique as it is introduced. One manager may describe poor communications as being the root cause of all his problems and will ask for expert advice on communication systems. An enthusiastic manager may see his problems arising from poor staff relations and ask a sociologist to provide techniques for improving them. Alternatively a manager may dismiss all management techniques as useless gimmicks and loudly state his preference for the 'good old rough and ready methods' of settling problems.

If managers are to avoid falling into any of these pitfalls they must understand both the capabilities and the limitations of the various management techniques and be prepared to show a healthy scepticism for any technique that is described as being able to solve all managerial problems. A manager who understands the principles, purpose and limitations of work study will make better use of it than one who does not.

With these provisos in mind the following description sets out the major techniques which are being gathered into management service departments. There is no monopoly on these techniques and managers may find a use for them possibly in a simplified form, or for the concept which lies behind them in the running of their own department. What is certain is that hospital managers will make increasing use of the management service departments to help them in the running of the hospital. This means that managerial decisions involving the pathology department will be taken on the advice and with the support of management services skills. This is a sound reason—even though it is a defensive one— why managers should understand managerial techniques and what they involve.

WORK STUDY

Work study aims to analyse performance in an unbiased manner and to arrange the information collected in such a way as to enable it to be studied to see if the best use is being made of resources. This is a much-maligned and misunderstood subject because of the way in which the term 'work study' is used in the industrial field. While large complex studies have to be carried out by qualified work-study staff, managers can themselves easily and usefully use many of the techniques of observation and presentation to look at the performance of their own department. The analysis of the information is no more difficult than many of the problems in medical laboratory technology. The following descriptions are based on the British Standards Institute Glossary of Terms in Work Study No. 3138 (1962).

Work study covers two main topics, Work Measurement and Method Study. Work measurement is the study to establish how long it takes a qualified worker to do a specified job at a defined level of performance. Method Study is the systematic recording and critical analysis of existing and proposed ways of doing work as a means of developing and applying easier and more effective methods and reducing costs. Examples of both of these techniques are described in the Hospital Services O & M Report No. 10 (1967).

Method Study

Four techniques are commonly used in method study:

(1) Flow process charts which set out the sequence of a procedure by recording all the events under review using appropriate symbols. These charts can be used to record worker material or equipment used in any particular process. An interesting example was described in a Report on Data Processing in Clinical Pathology in the *Journal of Clinical Pathology*, 1968. The authors made the following comments:

> In constructing a flow chart one inevitably finds oneself not only asking what exactly goes on but why and it is the necessity for clear thinking that makes construction of a flow process chart so valuable a discipline.

(2) Multiple activity charts show the activities of more than one worker or machine with a common time-scale to show their interrelationship. This enables related activities to be programmed together to avoid delays and bottle-necks in practise by their being out of gear.

(3) Flow diagrams or models show location, on a scale model, of specific activities carried out and the routes followed by workers, material and equipment in their execution. This is a useful technique to help in siting laboratories within a department or equipment within a laboratory. It will clearly identify overcrowded areas and at the same time remedies will be a lot more obvious.

(4) Activity sampling—a technique in which a large number of instantaneous observations are made over a period of time on a group of workers. Each observation records what is actually happening at that instant of time and the percentage of observation recorded for a particular activity is a measure of the percentage of time during which that activity is carried out. This technique can be used to estimate how much time technical staff spend on technical and non-technical duties. Observations could be made every hour during the working day for a week or two and would record whether the technician was doing technical or non-technical work. The timing and number of observations is related to the degree of precision required, being subject to the variations of random distribution. The total number of observations are then added and each group expressed as a percentage of this total.

Every O & M team insists that they do not want to become involved in studies leading to a reduction in staff as they would never be trusted by staff again—and there appears to be no evidence against this view. However O & M teams are abused in other ways. They are sometimes called in by the H.M.C. which is unable to implement a change desirable or otherwise. They ask the O & M team to make a study and then piously press through the recommendations (providing it agrees with their views) as being what the Regional Board O & M team recommends; the implication is that there is some connection between Regional Board policy and the findings of their O & M team. These examples of using O & M reports to prop up weak management are not uncommon.

Another disadvantage is that departmental managers tend to get left to one side during the search for a solution, following O & M Studies. Alternatively the team, because of their greater experience, may have found a suitable solution to a particular problem from previous studies and presented it extremely persuasively. In either case the manager is 'passing the buck' by tending to use the team as a crutch to prop himself up in a difficult situation instead of making at least the major part of any decision himself, having seen all the facts and listened to experienced people.

Probably the major shortcomings of O & M studies is that they describe the best way of doing a job but do not judge whether or not the job ought to be done. A study could recommend the best way of organizing the estimation of serum irons in terms of staff reagents and equipment but what it does not do is to say whether serum iron estimations should be done or not. There are many studies on the internal organization of pathology departments but none to identify their main purpose or objective. O & M teams seem to be better at analysis than synthesis. They are able to analyse work situations with considerable success but they are not able to synthesize working solutions with equal success. This may be for reasons beyond their control which they have to accept as limitations.

OPERATIONAL RESEARCH

Operational research is the attack of modern science on complex problems arising in the direction and management of large systems of men, machines, materials and money in any organization. Its distinctive approach is to develop scientific models of systems, incorporating measurement of factors such as chance and risk, with which to predict and compare the outcome of alternative decisions, strategies or controls. The purpose is to help management determine its policy and actions scientifically. New practices—

such as a new way of dealing with the collection of specimens—are more difficult to introduce as there is not usually a best way and a choice has to be made between several possible methods. Experience is a slow way of deciding how to choose the best method or how to make the best use of scarce resources.

War-time experience in finding or trying to find the best solution to military and logistic problems gave rise to the term 'operational research'. The method is one well known to technicians and scientists—that of first hypothesizing, then experimenting and testing the hypothesis. There are a large number of problems which can be expressed in the form of a diagram or model showing several different parameters. Staff in biochemistry laboratories will be familiar with this approach in the nomograms used in the Astrup methods for estimating blood pH and Pco_2 from a nomogram showing several parameters. Models can be either physical or, more commonly, mathematical. Their common characteristic is in being able to show all the variables in quantitative terms, so that the effect of change in one parameter can easily be predicted for another parameter.

An example of this has been published by the Oxford Regional Hospital Board Operational Research Unit in a paper entitled 'Optimum Purchasing Policy' (1962). This paper gives a general account of the method for deriving optimum order quantities and minimum stock levels. It considers the preliminary enquiries necessary to provide the basic data and gives examples of the various types of calculations encountered.

Revans (1965) claims that operational research shows that despite the random nature of the task of the manager, there exists a framework for treating many of his problems. Operational research recognizes that at all stages of the preparation of management decisions and in attempts to put these decisions into practice the operational research man is only able to forecast what is likely to happen. He does no more and claims to do no more than to estimate with less error than could be estimated in any other way what is likely to follow from any particular assumption and course of action.

There are a number of techniques commonly used in operational research which will be briefly mentioned. 'Network analysis' or 'system analysis' is an analytical technique used to calculate changes in output of an operation resulting from specified changes in input. It can also be used for managerial control of complex organizations. The general approach is that of viewing a problem or situation in its entirety with all its ramifications. The various forms of it—Programme Evaluation and Review Techniques (PERT), and Critical Path Analysis—have been widely used in scheduling work in industry.

CRITICAL PATH ANALYSIS

This analysis is generally considered to be a complicated procedure but it is not difficult to perform and it is as suitable for small tasks, such as setting up a cytology service, as it is for large tasks, such as building a hospital. The first step is to list in sequence, all the jobs that have to be done to complete such a task as setting up a cytology service. The second step is to express these jobs diagrammatically in the form of a network using an arrow to indicate activity and circles to represent the beginning or end of an activity (a node) (*see Figure 5*).

The diagram is drawn from left to right and the nodes numbered for identification. Once the diagram is complete an estimate is made of the time for each activity (in this case in days) and this entered on the diagram. The final phase is to analyse the diagram and isolate the sequence of events which takes the longest time. This sequence is the critical path and is the minimum time in which the task can be completed. In the example shown the critical path is marked and the minimum time for completion is 166 days. Activities not in the critical path will have spare time or 'float'—for example, such tasks as the designing and ordering of request forms. The amount of 'float' which can be permitted for non-critical activities can be readily estimated. If the critical path time and float times are tabulated this will provide a useful control as the jobs are being carried out. This technique can be used for many tasks in pathology departments. Revans in *Science and the Manager,* 1965 makes the analogy that a manager is like a lock-keeper controlling the flow of a river. The manager in a pathology department attempts to control the flow of reports or information from his department by moving a technician from one laboratory to another which is overworked or by putting more equipment into a particular laboratory. Revans states that the manager in charge of any flow system (and this would include those in pathology departments) needs to distinguish four major classes of decisions which are profusely illustrated in the literature of both operational research and sociology.

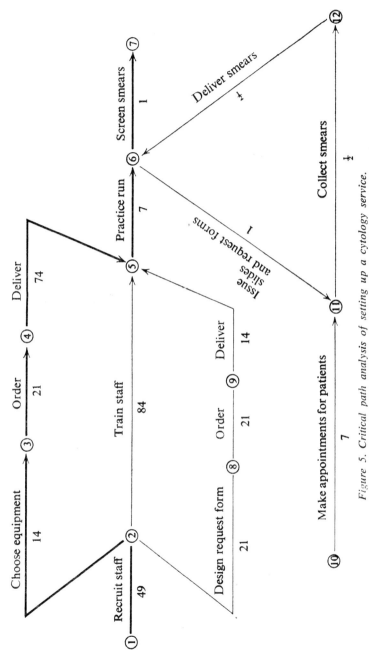

Figure 5. *Critical path analysis of setting up a cytology service.*

91

Classes of Decision

(1) There are decisions about items waiting for service when demand is greater than capacity. For example: how many technicians are required to perform a variable daily number of blood counts?; or how many staff must collect venous specimens of blood in an antenatal clinic to avoid patients waiting for more than a few minutes? (Queuing theories have useful applications in this sort of situation.) Again should laboratories be staffed to meet an average or the maximum work-load?

(2) Other types of decision are those concerning replacement in a flow system. This sort of decision crops up in pathology departments with an autoanalyser and similar automated equipment. The problem here may be to decide when is the best time to interrupt the system to replace a certain part and once the system has been stopped if it is worth replacing any other parts which appear to be in good condition but are equally old. Some attempt to reduce the maintenance costs of autoanalyser equipment could be made in this way.

(3) A third type of decision concerns allocation of resources. For instance with the resources available to a pathology department is it better to distribute the work among small teams or allocate it to larger teams?

(4) Finally, decisions are called for regarding spares and the amount of working material to be held in stock. This question is becoming increasingly important to departmental managers as the cost both of equipment and of essential spares increases. As stocks held in pathology departments are tying up large sums of money it is important that personnel should understand the basic principles of inventory control.

Input–Output Analysis

Another technique used in operational analysis is input–output analysis. This may be defined as a technique for describing in quantitative terms, the transaction which takes place during a specified period between a number of entities which are capable of making bilateral transactions between themselves (Redfurn, 1967). This technique can be applied to problems of producing qualified technicians by counting the number of students recruited over a certain period of years and the number of qualified staff produced. This input–output analysis will enable a manager to assess how many students will have to be recruited over, say, the next five years to produce the number of qualified technicians required. It would also help in the understanding of such problems as choosing between recruiting more staff or investing in more automated equipment to cope with increasing work-loads.

Cost Effectiveness

Cost effectiveness is a technique for comparing the cost of various alternative plans with their effectiveness. In trying to decide the best sort of staff to recruit, several alternatives can be considered. Each plan is considered in detail and an assessment of the cost made. This enables a close comparison to be made between the alternative programmes in terms of effectiveness and cost by systematically relating the different ranges of staff—graduate technician and assistant—to the sort of service that they could provide to meet clinicians' needs.

Cost Benefit Ratios

Cost benefit ratios use a similar technique to that of cost effectiveness in which a systematic study is made of the benefits derived from the investment of resources in different ways. It has been estimated to cost £220 to detect and treat a case of early carcinoma of the cervix for which the treatment is cheap; that of detecting and treating a case of invasive cervical carcinoma is estimated to be £650. These facts will assist in making decisions about investing in laboratory programmes for screening healthy populations. As the integration of hospitals, general practitioners and local authority work takes place laboratory directors and managers will be faced with many difficult problems in allocating their limited resources between these three areas and here the cost benefit ratios technique could be valuable.

The single theme which runs through all these techniques is the process of decision making, and managers should understand something about this process. Several steps can be identified in making a decision. The first is to define the problem clearly and to make sure that it is the basic problem and not simply a symptom arising from it. The second step is to discover and analyse alternative solutions. This is then followed by consideration of the anticipated results of the various solutions and the assessment of the best and worst of them. The decision itself is the actual choosing of one of the alternatives and this is followed by its implementation. Finally there is a check on whether the action decided upon is producing the anticipated result. All these steps are involved in any successful decision though they may not be taken consciously.

93

If any of the steps is omitted then the chances of successful implementation are reduced. If a symptom is mistaken for the main problem treatment of the symptom will not cure the problem though it may make life easier for a time.

Forecasting

A technique which many managers use is forecasting. In the simplest sense this means measuring past performance and extrapolating into the future. This is certainly better than nothing as it will avoid any gross underestimate or overestimate. It is frequently used to prove a case for more resources by slanting the evidence to over-forecast demand. This is likely to be less common in future as it becomes more easy to detect over-forecasting by improved methods of measuring performance.

Forecasting can be improved by a number of techniques described in two Monographs (Nos. 1 and 2) produced by I.C.I. (in 1962 and 1964 respectively). The use of Holt's Method for short-term forecasting is recommended using a modified seven-month moving average which should help to improve the accuracy of forecasting The authors state:

> Since Holt's method and similar methods of forecasting involve the projection of the trends of past demand into the future, it is important to ensure at the outset that past data are reliable and comparable in that no major change of markets or customers has occurred. Also, if possible that they relate to true demand and not merely to available supply.

This raises an interesting point in relation to demands for increased investment in pathology departments in which annual increases in numbers of requests are produced as justification for such increase. It would be equally true to say that the increased number of requests which have been processed simply reflects an increased capacity for processing requests. Alternatively one of Parkinson's Laws could apply—that the work will fill the time allotted to it. Some measure should be made of the number of requests turned down in order to estimate the unfulfilled demand from clinicians; or possibly the delay in processing requests.

CONTROL SYSTEMS

There are a number of control systems which can be helpful in pathology departments if sensibly applied, with full understanding of the purpose and limitations of control systems in general. Any such system necessitates some sort of target being set and a flow of information showing whether or not that target or objective is being achieved.

Quality Control

This form of control is widely used in biochemistry laboratories and perhaps to a lesser extent in haematology laboratories. It is based on the method in the A.C.P. Broadsheet No. 30 (1964) which describes the principles of the method as applied to technical estimations. Quality control can equally well be applied to screening cytology smears and a method has been described by Weaver and Puente (1964) which can maintain standards of efficiency while detecting and confirming positive smears without a great deal of effort. Quality control has much wider applications than simply technical work. It can be introduced at the final stage before the reports are sent out to clinicians and a 10 per cent sample could be taken to check the quality of such reports apart from their technical information: for example, for legibility, correct destination, time taken to process request and so on, thus assessing the overall performance of the department. Similar methods could be introduced in recruiting staff by checking methods of selecting students against their performance over the next three years. This will enable criteria of selection to be checked and reset if necessary.

Budgetary Control

Budgetary control assumes that a target has been set for cost either as total cost or unit cost. Information is collected and analysed with a view to correcting any overshooting of the target. The difficulty with budgetary control is that most costing figures take so long to prepare that it is too late to correct any overshooting. However this snag is likely to be overcome in the near future with increasing use of computers to produce accounting information. Unit cost figures can be used to compare the performance of the department year by year. The system was never designed to compare the cost of different departments. The national or regional average unit cost is included to show average increases from one year to the next. This control system will be increasingly used in the future.

Inventory Control

As previously mentioned inventories will become increasingly necessary as the value of stocks and spares held increases. It was not a great sum when pathology departments were relatively small but now that some departments have an annual budget of over £100,000 the value of stocks and spares must be mounting up. A figure will have to be set for individual pieces of automated equipment costing £30,000–£40,000. Spares to the figure of ten per cent of the total cost would involve £3,000–£4,000 being tied up doing nothing apart from depreciating.

Disadvantages of Controls

As suggested earlier controls are not without disadvantages. Information can be expensive to collect. The type of control system tends to influence management policy. This can be seen in the department which undertakes a large number of simple tests in order to keep its unit cost down and its technician–request ratio up. Control information is for the use of the department not to enable higher authorities to call them to order. Controls such as unit cost can also be used as a smoke screen to hide indifference. Management policy is centred, metaphorically speaking, on keeping in the centre of the league table as far as unit cost is concerned and avoiding awkward questions; regrettably in the end this could become more important than providing an effective service.

ERGONOMICS

Broadly speaking ergonomics is the science of fitting the job to the worker using techniques from a number of fields. It is the study of all the factors which influence the physical and psychological relationship between man and his work. It is concerned with matters as diverse as the height of a chair, accessibility of controls, humidity in a laundry and suitability of a task for a man of 60 years of age. In all cases ergonomics asks the question: are the conditions the most suitable for the staff who will be affected by them? As a matter of practical interest ergonomics has already produced many ideas which, if used in pathology departments, could decrease fatigue, lower staff turnover, reduce accidents and provide greater work satisfaction. The Department of Scientific and Industrial Research have published a series of pamphlets 'Ergonomics in Industry' (1964), as a guide to the application of ergonomic research.

Problems arise whenever it is necessary to read dials or gauges on instruments. Evidence suggests that more mistakes are made in reading some sorts of dials than others depending on the position of the dials and the design of the pointer. Lighting in pathology departments is generally inadequate judging by the number of extra lights which are placed on benches. The Hospital Building Notes for Pathology Departments (Ministry of Health, 1965) call for 25 lumens per square foot at floor level in laboratories. This is insufficient for many activities carried out on benches, though no investigations have been made into optimum lighting intensities. Noise can be unpleasant in terms of intensity and pitch. Equipment such as high speed centrifuges produces considerable noise which could result in some degree of deafness among staff.

In the past equipment has been relatively small and has not called for any great effort from staff using it. The one exception to this was perhaps the microscope which, unless carefully positioned, can cause discomfort to the user. Observation of staff using microscopes reveals how uncomfortable many of them are. Either the bench is too high or the chairs too high for the technician to put his feet on the ground, arms are not supported and the general picture is not one of comfort and relaxation. Now that the equipment is larger and more expensive it is more urgent to consider the design in relation to the worker so that both are working at optimum efficiency.

CHAPTER 6

STAFF MANAGEMENT

INTRODUCTION

Staff are the most important and expensive item in pathology departments, salaries being over 70 per cent of the total expenditure. Recruiting and training them takes up a great deal of time and the results are very uncertain. It is still left mainly to chance and this results in the familiar progression from one staff crisis to another. Some departments attempt a more positive policy but are rarely successful because their approach is not based on factual information. This situation is more difficult than ever today and there is an urgent need for a systematic approach to the problem, such as collecting and analysing facts about recruitment, training and utilization of staff. After such analysis a long-term plan for staffing can be formulated. This approach has become more common in planning for money and equipment in recent years and it is difficult to understand why it has not been used to plan staff requirements in pathology departments.

The general feeling is that departments have managed in the past and they will manage in the future. There are a number of reasons why this is over-optimistic. Money will be scarce in the N.H.S. for many years to come and there will be constant pressure to improve the performance of pathology departments. The recruitment of technicians will be affected by the introduction of the National Certificate system; training is likely to be centralized. Recommendations for the post-qualification training of pathologists and biochemists is likely to alter the recruitment pattern particularly in small departments. Automation will change staffing patterns and alter the present ratio of technicians to technologists. Change in the existing tripartite arrangement of the N.H.S. and in medical practice will in turn bring changes in the type of service pathology departments have to provide—such as the screening of the healthy population.

Chief technicians and pathologists do not count their individual technical staff as assets in the same way as they value laboratory equipment or buildings. They speak of taking on students or technicians as they might hire a new pH meter. If this were to break down it could be replaced the next day without extra cost. If, however, the complete technical staff left a department, the cost of replacing them with an equally effective staff would be enormous. Many industrial companies have estimated the replacement cost of staff to be several times their annual salary, which gives the technical staff an asset value considerably greater than that of all the other assets in the department, the annual salary bill being analagous to running costs. No manager would survive if he used equipment of equivalent value so wastefully as he tends to use his staff.

STAFF PLANNING

The essence of staff planning is to decide the number and grades of staff required for the next five or ten years and the number likely to be available from existing trainees or that can be recruited. Then a comparison is made between predicted demand and supply; differences can then be assessed and finally a plan formulated to recruit and train suitable people. Before it is possible to forecast the number of staff required, information has to be collected about the existing staff, numbers recruited, how long they have been employed, how many qualified, and reasons for leaving when they do so. This information should be set out in the form of tables and graphs to aid analysis.

STAFF UTILIZATION

Some indication of how staff are used can be deduced from examination of the annual reports of the Chief Medical Officer of the Ministry of Health (1958–1966) (*see* Table 1). The national average of requests per technician was 3,560 in 1960, it had risen to 4,240 in 1964 and dropped to 4,070 by 1966. These ratios are relatively crude but give a good indication of trends. They tend to over-simplify the problems in any one particular pathology department in which a more detailed analysis is required. The ratio of qualified to unqualified technicians showed an abrupt alteration in 1963 (Table 4, page 18). This was not due to any change in policy or a preconceived plan. It was due to the replacement by students of the large number of qualified technicians who left the N.H.S. at that time because of low salaries.

The Hospital Services O & M Report No. 10 (1967) sets out a convenient method of analysing technical work and the percentage of time technicians spend on it and gives a formula for assessing how effectively technicians time is utilized. It lists the findings of a number of studies of work in various departments and sets out some useful average values for distribution of tests in laboratories and average times taken to do each test. The report points out that only 50 per cent of technicians' time is spent doing technical work. Bennett (1967) found that students and junior technicians spent 25 per cent of their time doing work which required no training and could be undertaken by other grades of staff, such as laboratory assistants. Experience with automated equipment indicates that technicians using it spend 30 per cent of their time handling report or request forms. The general consensus of opinion among technicians is that the bulk of the routine work has been done by junior technicians for many years because of force of circumstances. So far no studies have been made of the work done by biochemists and pathologists and this will make it difficult to make any sort of forecast at present about future requirements of these grades of staff.

STAFF FORECASTING

The demand for staff over the next five- to ten-year period can be predicted by projecting the increase in the number of requests over the ten years from 1957 into the next ten years (*Figure 6*) and calculating from the present request–technician ratio the number of extra staff required each year as in Table 8. This will enable a recruiting programme to be drawn up and will also serve as part of the forward planning of non-recurring costs. It should be noted that this will only indicate the number of pairs of hands required and not the grades of staff. The same exercise can be undertaken for each laboratory in a department, giving a more precise forecast by including the various grades of staff that will be required over the ten-year period. When forecasting staff demand, it is necessary to consider the number of days worked annually by technicians. Since 1962 there has been a progressive reduction in the number of working days per year. In 1962 when a department took advantage of the new regulations permitting day-release for student technicians it lost 14 per cent of students' annual working days. Table 9 has been drawn up to show the decrease in days per working year calculated as a percentage loss of total staff working days, using as an example a department with a staff of 32 made up of 12 qualified staff, 8 juniors and 12 students.

100

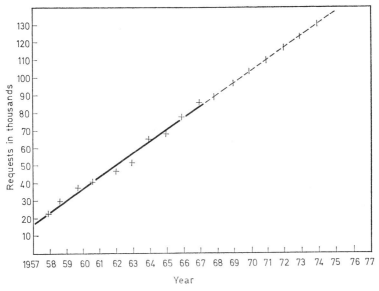

Figure 6. Work forecast.

TABLE 8

Year	No. of requests	Increase in staff	Total staff	Requests/technician
1957	18,892	—	10	1,900
1958	23,959	2	12	2,000
1959	28,077	—	12	2,300
1960	36,093	1	13	2,800
1961	41,744	—	13	3,200
1962	43,369	2	15	2,900
1963	46,735	—	15	3,100
1964	61,100	1	16	3,800
1965	68,420	1	17	4,000
1966	77,121	3	20	3,850
1967	82,321	1	21	3,900
1968	90,000	2	23	3,900
1969	98,000	2	25	3,900
1970	103,000	2	27	3,900
1971	110,000	1	28	3,900
1972	115,000	2	30	3,900
1973	121,000	1	31	3,900
1974	130,000	2	33	3,900

TABLE 9

Year	New regulation	Percentage of work days lost	Technician equivalent	National average request/technician ratio
1961	—	—	—	3,729
1962	Day-release	5	$1\frac{1}{2}$	3,820
1963	—	—	—	4,000
1964	Increased holiday for 18–21 year group	<1	1/18	4,200
1964	Working hours reduced 39–38 per week	2.5	$\frac{3}{4}$	4,200
1965	—	—	—	4,070
1966	Block-release	1	$\frac{1}{3}$	4,070

The 1 per cent loss of work days incurred for block-release in 1966 assumes that the department had implemented day-release, in 1962. The total percentage loss for this period amounts to approximately 10 per cent and represents the work of three technicians. It is difficult to understand recent claims that a 25 per cent increase of staff would be required to allow students to attend block-release courses. This progressive reduction in working hours can be expected to continue.

To forecast the supply of staff for the same period it is possible to estimate those likely to stay in such posts over the next ten years and the number of students who are expected to qualify in the same period. The latter can be calculated from previous records of the number of new students employed, the number passing the I.M.L.T. Intermediate and Final examinations and those qualified technicians still employed. This will indicate the number of qualified technicians likely to result from employing a certain number of new students. For example, if 60 students were recruited during the last ten years and 20 are now qualified and still working in the department, it can reasonably be assumed that this can be repeated in the next ten-year period. Thus if 40 qualified technicians are required, recruitment will have to reach twice the previous rate of 60 per year.

A similar forecast has to be made about the probable supply of new recruits in pathology departments. This problem will present itself differently in a large industrial town in comparison to a small town where opportunity for employment in scientific establishments is low. Qualified staff and university graduates are more likely to work in big centres near teaching hospitals. More employers are looking for school leavers with either O-level or A-level passes, who are interested in science.

It is estimated that the number of school leavers at O-level will fall by 20 per cent from 1965 to 1970. It is gloomily assumed that the majority staying on to attempt A-levels are bound for universities but evidence shows that only 50 per cent of those obtaining two A-level passes will reach university; 7 per cent will go to Colleges of Advanced Technology or Technical Colleges. Approximately 20 per cent will go straight into employment and this figure is likely to increase. Taking one subject in the 1965 A-level examination; 32,000 sat the chemistry paper, 70 per cent passed and of these only half went on to university.

On the other hand, many Comprehensive and some Secondary Modern Schools are now teaching pupils to the level of the Certificate of Secondary Education (C.S.E.), grade 1 being equivalent to a pass at O-level. Many pupils are leaving these schools with four C.S.E. grade 1 passes and are eligible for O.N.C. courses. There is not really a shortage of suitable school leavers as in parts of the country some have difficulty in finding jobs. The shortage is often an artificial one created by the unwillingness of pathology departments to put effort into recruiting or to look for alternative sources of recruitment.

It has already been noted that in 1962 the number of qualified technicians in the N.H.S. decreased by several hundred and in the same year over 500 passed their first I.M.L.T. Final Examination. In 1966 qualified technicians increased in the N.H.S. by 237, while 633 passed their I.M.L.T. Final Examination (Table 6, page 19). This suggests that there is not a shortage of technicians in the country, so it must be assumed that the N.H.S. is not willing to pay salaries sufficiently attractive to prevent them from being drawn away by other employers. It would also explain to some extent the amount of over-grading of technicians that exists today.

With regard to biochemists, the forecast seems to be that the present difficult position regarding recruiting them is not likely to improve. The shortage of medical manpower is likely to continue for the next ten years and although the present number of trainee pathologists is considered adequate to meet present needs, there is little possibility of rapidly expanding the number of consultant pathologists.

This assessment of future demand for and supply of staff will enable plans to be made for recruiting and training them. Where there is a large gap between predicted demand and supply, various actions to remedy this will have to be considered depending on the reason for the gap. It may be helpful to reduce the department's training commitments by recruiting clerical assistants to relieve technologists of their clerical work or laboratory assistants to relieve technicians of their non-technical work. Balancing recruitment into the three grades of student, junior and technician will maintain a better distribution of staff away at technical college at any one period. For example, rather than recruiting six students at once, it may be better to recruit four students with O-levels who enter the O.N.C. course and two with A-levels who can go straight into the H.N.C. course. Wastage of students in the first few years may be reduced by recruiting more men than women.

These plans should be such that the department will be able to provide the service needed by clinicians and reasonable career prospects for staff of all grades. They should also make the best use of the money that is likely to be available in future years.

Staff planning has to be carried out in the prevailing climate within the H.M.C., the Regional Board and the Ministry of Health. There are many factors which it is impossible to control, such as the money allocated to an H.M.C. by the Regional Board. Forecasting is made difficult by changes in policy by the Minister of Health, and by the future allocation of money which is influenced by the political situation as well as by the financial state of the nation. Deployment and training of staff is radically influenced by the professional bodies with their views on post-qualification training and by the Registration Boards. It is hard to assess how the attitudes of the professional groups in pathology departments will change. How will pathologists react to chief technicians as departmental managers, technicians to extended hours, or biochemists to the idea of providing a service for clinicians?

RECRUITMENT

Few departments have waiting lists of school leavers seeking to become student technicians and the majority are only too familiar with the problems of recruiting and retaining students. Causes are well known—poor response to advertisements, difficulties in selecting staff and poor educational standards of applicants. Departmental managers, in an effort to maintain a steady intake of good students, should give some thought to techniques of recruitment selection, induction and training as well as to the labour market from which it recruits staff.

It is not enough simply to place an advertisement in a local paper offering school leavers a career as a student technician with conditions of service as laid down by the Whitley Council, when it is quite likely that they have no idea at all what laboratory technicians do or what Whitley Council regulations are. Experience has shown that only one-third of applicants for students' vacancies come in response to advertisements in local papers. Some come as the result of interviews with Youth Employment Officers and others have heard about the job from friends. Rarely has the career been recommended by careers' masters in grammar schools. Enthusiastic chief technicians who attend careers conventions so often come up against this same problem—that pupils have never heard of the job. This can be tackled in a number of ways. Recruitment literature can be sent to careers' masters in all types of secondary schools; many a careers master in a Secondary Modern School would be grateful to be able to offer this sort of job to his brightest pupils. Visits to the department should be arranged for pupils in the first half of their fifth year when they are beginning seriously to consider choosing their career. A visit will be of little value, however, if a whole class attends for then it becomes a mere tour of 30 pupils round the department with only a few showing any interest. The better approach is to write to the headmaster asking him to advertise the visit among fifth-form pupils who are interested and in this way smaller groups, possibly collected from two or three schools, can be shown around the department, receive demonstrations and finally be given a talk on careers in Medical Technology. Admittedly, visits of this sort cost time and money but this investment will be repaid many times over if the level of applicants improves as a result.

Another hopeful method is to persuade science masters to invite senior technicians to attend the school and give technical demonstrations instead of the rather dull careers talk normally given. The A-level syllabus in Zoology and Botany includes much practical work which is part of the daily routine in pathology departments and could be of great assistance to science masters in preparing interesting demonstrations. Many of the microscopic preparations such as those of reticulocytes, buffy-coat layers or chromosome spreads, which are thrown away after they have been examined, would be considered invaluable by science masters.

When recruiting staff local conditions must be carefully studied and taken into consideration. Where a hospital is situated in a rural area the field of recruitment is limited because of the difficulties and cost of travelling more than ten miles to work. Under these circumstances, offers of accommodation in the hospital, if at all possible, will considerably widen the catchment area from which recruits can be drawn. Comparison of the records of a small number of departments clearly shows that students recruited at the end of the school year or early in the autumn have a lower drop-out rate than those recruited at other times of the year. Recruitment is not always possible then but it has much to recommend it even if it means bringing back qualified married women for a temporary period.

Finally, on the subject of recruiting, the Dainton Committee made the comment that: 'the reputation of the good employer is the most enduring career guidance system of all; employers must recognize their high responsibility for ensuring careers in science, engineering and technology are satisfying and therefore attractive to young people' (Enquiry into the flow of Candidates in Science and Technology into Higher Education H.M.S.O. Cmd 3541, 1968).

Selection

Since selection is a process of matching up people with available jobs, the first step must be to write a personnel specification describing the qualifications and characteristics needed if a person is to be successful in a particular job. This is best done by a systematic study of the job in question. As an example: a student technician has to enter an O.N.C. course so he must have four O-level passes; furthermore, he has to meet patients and therefore must have a reasonable appearance, a pleasant manner and be able to express himself well; he has to be able to accept the scientific discipline inherent in medical technology and be able to cope with work situations in which emergencies are common and the pressure of work is high; in the course of his daily work he must carry out estimations on blood, urine, faeces and other specimens and must therefore be able to cope with this aspect of the work.

The next step is to advertise the vacancy. The advertisement should announce the vacancy and how to apply but should not attempt to describe the job as this is part of the recruitment procedure. Timing should be related to publication of O-level examination results in the area. The vacancies should be published in local newspapers and sent to Youth Employment Officers and to headmasters well before the end of term. In response to enquiries, application forms should be sent out. This form is an instrument for collecting information, particularly that relating to qualifications, to decide who shall be interviewed and also to get facts on which to base the interview. The selection of applicants for the short list is made by checking qualifications against the job qualification. Standard application forms are usually designed for adults and are not really suitable for school leavers. It is an advantage to include a supplementary form with questions about activities at school other than academic studies. Once the short list has been drawn up, letters are sent to referees describing the post and enquiring about the character and ability of the applicant. Although references are potentially important, they are often biased or noncommittal and only constitute a negative check. Referees can be encouraged to be forthright by telling them the reference is confidential.

Interviewing

Successful interviews need a certain amount of preparatory work. Letters are sent out giving the date, place and time of the interview. If more than two or three applicants are being interviewed, the appointment times should be staggered to avoid them waiting, but adequate time should be allowed for the interview itself. The applicant should be given clear instructions as to where he should attend and someone should be detailed to meet him on arrival—probably the receptionist or the hall porter. A suitable room should be set aside for the interview where interruptions by other members of the staff or telephone calls are unlikely, for an interview is a private discussion and is less likely to be successful if interrupted.

Ideally, interviewing should be done by one person who is an expert but it is more common in practice to find it carried out by a panel consisting of the hospital secretary, pathologist and chief technician. It is advisable to keep the panel as small as possible so that the free flow of information from the applicant is not inhibited. If a department sends its students to a local technical college it is very helpful to have the head of the science department on the interview panel as this will ensure an expert view on the student's ability to follow the course. The biggest danger of panel interviews is that members tend to ask questions in no particular order and this frequently confuses the applicant. Before the interview it is necessary to determine exactly what the interview is trying to achieve. This can best be defined as a method of collecting facts from the applicant about himself to enable an assessment to be made for comparison with the job specification. For people with little experience of interviewing it is helpful to make a list of the questions to be asked and particular points to be raised relating to the facts on the application form. It may be necessary to collect from within the department information which may be asked for by applicants.

An assessment rating form should be designed, using some simple arrangement such as the Five Point Plan (Munro Fraser, 1965) to enable both a relatively unbiased assessment and a comparison between the applicants to be made. Before the interview it is necessary for the interviewer to understand and appreciate his own attitudes in assessing the characteristics of people generally. The appearance of school leavers must be judged against the current fashion of the age group and it must be accepted that long hair is quite usual, narrow trousers are standard wear and shoes are not likely to be those that either the pathologist or chief technician would choose to wear himself. When considering intelligence, it is important to look for the ability to think in abstract terms. Above-average intelligence is usually associated with special aptitudes, high scholastic achievement and good conversational ability. Interest in and membership of school societies can reveal quite a lot in the applicant, while his attitude to authority can be assessed by his reaction to the staff who taught him. It is more difficult to assess emotional stability but some idea can be gained from how objectively an applicant describes himself.

It is important to establish good *rapport* if worthwhile results are to be achieved at the interview. The applicant should first be introduced to the people in the room and asked to take a chair. The chairman of the panel should then start the interview either by describing the job or checking through some of the details on the application form so giving the applicant a chance to settle down and relax. From then on he should be encouraged to talk but never allowed to flounder, and long silences should be avoided. Questions should always require more than a 'yes' or 'no' as a reply and every effort must be made to avoid judging or criticizing any comment from the applicant. It is necessary to learn to listen. The interviewing should not be rushed but should always be kept to the point and under the control of the interviewer. The meaning of a question is closely associated with the educational and emotional background of the questioner so questions to young applicants must be clear and readily understandable. The facial expressions, gestures and tone of voice of the applicant should be noted as they also convey meaning. Finally, the applicant should be asked if he would take the job if it were offered to him. The interview should be closed courteously and the applicant thanked for attending.

As soon as the interview has been completed the rating form should be filled in, in an attempt to assess the character and record any relevant facts. When all the interviews have been completed, it is then possible to match up the assessment forms with the job specification. A choice is made from those which make the best match. The successful applicants should be called in one by one and offered the job and their acceptance should be obtained. The remainder of the applicants should be called in and told they have been unsuccessful and thanked for attending the interview. Arrangements should then be made for paying travelling expenses for applicants.

Interviewing is an acquired skill presenting a number of aspects so that little formal advice can be offered apart from stressing the value both of systematic approach and helpful information about techniques. The interviewer can himself develop his skills by practical and critical examination of his failures and successes. No one likes to think that he cannot interview successfully for this implies that he cannot judge people, encourage them to talk freely and understand their point of view. Interviewing young people is particularly difficult because of their limited experience, and lack of confidence makes it even more difficult to establish *rapport* during the interview. This calls for a light touch particularly in the line of questioning. A straight question about hobbies will not get very far. Knowledge both of the sort of pursuits local young people follow and also of the facilities available in the locality is necessary.

Recruitment of qualified staff should be carried out in much the same way but paying more attention to the reasons for the applicant wanting the job, as this is important in relation to qualified staff. A job analysis should be carried out and it should form the basis of the job specification detailing the training, qualifications and characteristics sought in the person most suitable for the post. A Five Point Plan similar to that of Munro Fraser (1962) should be used as a guide and the same process of matching assessment of applicants with job specification. Much time can be wasted in interviews by repeating the job description to every applicant at the beginning of each interview and to avoid this a detailed job description should be sent out with each application form.

In practice many interviews consist of an untrained employer talking generalities about a job which he has not analysed to a would-be employee about whom he knows little and then deciding whether or not to offer him the job. The applicant's impression of the department as well as the job for which he has applied are coloured by the way in which the interview is conducted. The interview is a two-way affair. Information should flow in both directions as a separate assessment is made by both parties. The applicant will have formed an impression about the interview, about who personifies the company and about the way in which the job was described. On such evidence he will make up his mind whether or not to accept the job if it were offered to him.

Induction

Changing from school to work creates serious problems for young people. To summarize the relevant observations made by Carter in his book *Into Work*, 1966: 'The pace is faster at work than at school, the hours longer, meal breaks and holidays are shorter and often there is a six-day week instead of the five-day week of school. Students have commented that it takes months to forget the atmosphere of school and such things as prefects and teachers. Standards of behaviour are different in the adult world of work and staff so often assume that new students are automatically aware of this. These problems are more acute for the less mature boys and girls. Pathology departments are complex and hospitals tend to be large and impersonal so that it takes time to become familiar with them. Students will work enthusiastically if they have a broad idea of the purpose of the department, particularly the section they are to work in. Becoming a student means entering a group and seeking a social satisfaction which depends on being accepted as a member of that group. Students are very concerned about making fools of themselves but may be too timid to ask questions to avoid this. There is ample evidence in the Crowther Report (1959, 1960) and elsewhere that induction courses are worthwhile and reduce the turnover among student technicians.

The following induction course has been successfully used for several years. On arrival in the department the new student is met by the chief technician who explains briefly the organization of the department and such general things as hours of work, meal breaks and the necessity for understanding the confidential nature of the work. The student is then taken to the hospital administrative office and the formalities of signing on are completed. At intervals during the first week the new student is given short talks on the profession of medical technology by the chief technician, the technician–patient relationship by a pathologist and the social aspect of medicine by the medical social worker. The sister tutor arranges visits to wards and out-patient departments and explains the various ranks of nursing staff and ward etiquette. One senior technician from each laboratory explains the function and set-up of his particular laboratory. A final meeting is then held to cover such things as safety and laboratory hazards and any other questions which may have arisen during the first week, and to make sure that the student has understood the bulk of the information that has been given to him. These induction lectures not only help the student to settle down and understand a little of the pathology department but it also gives him an opportunity to meet some of the senior people in the hospital and certainly for the pathologist to meet the new student. Ideally, the process of induction should be continued into general studies in the O.N.C. course; students should be encouraged to understand more about adults in the working situation and why people go to work and the behaviour of informal groups at work. It is then up to the senior under whom they are to work not only to continue the induction and make quite sure that the student knows to whom he should go if in difficulties but generally to help him to settle down.

EDUCATION AND TRAINING

Only pre-qualification training is provided for technicians and it consists of each student spending six months in each of the four laboratories in the department. It is virtually impossible to arrange that a student working in a laboratory is doing the same sort of work as he is studying at the technical college. The smaller the department, the more traumatic is the change-over period when students move from one laboratory to another. These departments will have to examine their student training and seriously consider alternatives, however unpalatable, such as employing laboratory assistants in place of students or exchanging students with a larger department.

Large departments cannot avoid training and 'rotating' students but the task can be made less onerous. The departmental manager must keep records of each student's training and his progress round the laboratories and plan future movement, keeping technicians in charge of laboratories informed well in advance of the actual move. The manager can keep a balance between the groups of students in training by recruiting at different levels. One person

111

in each laboratory must be made responsible for supervising student training. Each student should be given a written programme of the techniques he is expected to learn during his stay in each laboratory. Only the techniques in everyday use should be included in this programme for it is unfair to expect senior staff to put up special demonstrations. The student should keep a written record of each technique as he learns it, thus enabling the senior technician to check his progress and comprehension.

Pathology departments provide post-qualification training for pathologists, biochemists and technicians for higher qualifications specified by their respective professional bodies. These higher qualifications are necessary for promotion but only partly cover the range of skills used by the three groups. Analysis of the activities in pathology departments has already identified three major jobs, director, manager and technologist, none being covered by the present training for higher qualifications. No amount of exhortation will induce any of the three professional bodies to provide this type of training and indeed it is doubtful if it is their responsibility. Training in management should be undertaken by the employer. At present it is provided by some Regional Hospital Boards and such bodies as the King Edward VII Hospital Fund for London. The courses in the past have tended to be more concerned with theory and managerial techniques than with the skills used in day-to-day activities.

This then is the training commitment of a pathology department. The three professional groups are trained mainly by exposing them to the influence of experienced staff working on the bench. Experience and research in industry show quite clearly that training by 'exposure' is slow, expensive and very boring for the trainee. Finally, it must be stressed that education is a process of creating perception, judgment and training; indeed the acquisition of skills is a continuous process and not one that is complete when a qualification is obtained. Revans (1965) has drawn attention to the serious deficiencies of technical education in this country.

PROMOTION POLICY

Whitley Council Regulations state that the grading of technicians is related to the number of staff they supervise and hence the amount of responsibility they take. The regulations include an escape clause—which is widely used—whereby technicians can be promoted if they are engaged on individual work of special responsibility and skill. Some pathologists seem to use promotion as a reward for long service, for being a 'blue-eyed boy' or to retain a skilled and, seemingly, irreplaceable technician. These sort of reasons invariably cause resentment among staff who are not rewarded in this way. Technicians have come to expect promotion not only to be related to the number of staff supervised but also to obtaining a qualification. Until recently junior technicians expected automatic promotion to technician grade on qualifying.

The traditional promotion pattern has been distorted by increasing automation which enables a senior technician with five staff to turn out two or three times as much work as before. On the other hand histology laboratories have expanded more slowly than the others and promotion in this department is also slower. The shortage of qualified staff inside the N.H.S. has increased inter-departmental competition for staff and it seems easier to upgrade a technician to retain him than to get an increase in establishment. Over-grading of technicians in this way is a defensive reaction against other employers who are willing to offer higher salaries to technicians. These reasons make it difficult to institute a rational and planned promotion policy. Senior pathologists in some of the larger departments have drifted away from any sort of promotion policy and both technicians and pathologists are confused.

Appraisal of Staff Performance

Pathologists and chief technicans would readily agree that an important part of their job is to develop methods and equipment but few would agree that it is more important to develop staff. They tend to accept ineffective staff and are extremely reluctant to sack them or even to pass them over for promotion. This lack of action is often excused by dismissing it as the person having a personality problem and assuming that this cannot be altered. People can do so much more than mere mechanical work and have considerable latent ability as well as enthusiasm which can be developed. Any staff development scheme requires appraisal of their performance rather than of their personality.

Staff appraisal schemes have been successfully used in the Civil Service for many years and have been recently introduced for hospital administrative staff. This is not an easy technique to introduce particularly if it is taken to mean appraising people instead of their performance. There are many advantages to be gained from the introduction of staff and performance appraisal into pathology departments for it would help in creating a promotion policy based on facts rather than on impressions and feelings. It

113

would also help to orientate the attention of directors and managers towards one of their major jobs—that of developing staff, the department's most expensive asset.

HEALTH, SAFETY AND WELFARE

Health

The Reid Report of 1956 showed that precautions to avoid T.B. infections by staff working in bacteriology laboratories were inadequate and made a number of recommendations, but a survey made a few years afterwards by the Association of Scientific Workers (1965) showed that the recommendations were not being widely implemented and cases are still being reported. Health should be of vital concern to the top team in pathology. Any efficient chief technician will have some of his equipment under a service contract but may not be prepared to take the same amount of trouble with the health of his staff. Experience has shown that the normal medical check required on employment of new staff is of limited value. Such defects as low haemoglobin levels in females, colour-blindness and defective vision are more common than is generally supposed and should be looked for. Among senior staff it is worthwhile to keep a look out for more obvious conditions ranging from allergic skin conditions to such things as flat feet—a condition which accounted for one technician becoming bad tempered; both feet and temper improved rapidly with appropriate treatment!

Safety

Considering pathology departments are scientific establishments the risks that are taken with such things as electrical equipment and dangerous chemicals are quite astonishing. Highly poisonous chemicals are left on shelves and electrical wiring often leaves much to be desired. Supervising safety regulations should be laid down as being part of the duties of a technologist and it is up to him to ensure the health and safety of his staff. This should start with the introduction of new students and should go on as a continuous process. It is recommended that the dangers should be brought to the notice of staff and detailed precautions described to prevent accidents. This should cover such things as inflammable or dangerous vapours particularly in chromatography, or in histology laboratories, carcinogenic chemicals, radioactive isotopes and accidental bacteriological infections. Technologists should also be concerned with accident prevention; because accidents are relatively rare, precautions tend to be lax and small things overlooked. Accidents are never caused by single mistakes and there are invariably three or more contributory factors. If any one of these factors was absent the accident would probably never have occurred. A careful analysis of every accident should be undertaken to distinguish primary and contributory factors. Students should never be allowed to handle dangerous chemicals until they have been taught safety precautions.

Welfare

Welfare of staff in terms of their emotional well-being is a relatively unknown area in pathology departments, possibly because problems occurring in this area are considered inevitable and impossible to treat. Staff may have problems about their careers or training. New students coming into the department tend to go through severe reactions in the change from school to adult life and need to be handled with tact and perception if they are to settle down satisfactorily. Occasionally some will fail to become a member of an informal group and remain isolated and this always leads to abnormal behaviour. Problems of accommodation, disagreements with parents and boy or girl friends are likely to alter behaviour and working patterns of staff. Senior staff need to be aware of these problems and understand the alterations they are likely to produce. Punishment and threats are quite inappropriate and they call for tact, understanding, sympathy and a great deal of patience.

SUMMARY

Staff are the most important and expensive of all the resources in pathology departments. There are techniques for staff planning, utilization and forecasting which help to make the best use of staff, and aid in balancing future supply against demand. Recruitment, selection, induction and training are all vital activities and the manager's performance can be improved by using modern methods. It is also stressed that a more rational approach to promotion and staff appraisal can be made. Finally, staff health and welfare are important matters which should not be neglected. While this chapter deals primarily with technicians, much of what has been written applies equally to pathologists and biochemists.

CHAPTER 7

HUMAN PERSONALITY AND BEHAVIOUR AT WORK

INTRODUCTION

So far this book has been concerned with the organization of pathology departments and relevant managerial skills, all of which are impersonal, but this is not enough as many senior staff will have recognized. Reference has previously been made in Chapter 2 to the lack of understanding and trust between the three professional groups (in pathology departments) which reduces efficiency and makes some departments unhappy places in which to work. There may not be open conflict but frequently the staff express their feelings either by leaving for other jobs or by becoming indifferent and lacking in enthusiasm and commitment to the work. All three groups are primarily concerned with medicine and technology and often regard staff matters as a burden—indeed in some cases they may not even have a hand in selecting staff. The situation can hardly be made worse by looking at what motivates people to work and co-operate and what prevents them from doing this. Nor can it be a bad thing for director, manager and technologist to understand or learn to understand their own motives and what effect their behaviour has on other people. This chapter will consider some aspects of human behaviour and motivation, the characteristics of groups of people at work and the implications for directors, managers and technologists.

The fact that staff costs make up some 65–70 per cent of the total cost of running a department is another sound reason for learning more about human behaviour and work groups. If the handling of equipment is compared with the handling of staff some curious anomalies come to light. For example, a cell counter is selected with care, is checked for accuracy of performance every day, and is usually on a maintenance contract at regular intervals and handled by staff specially trained to use it. Any member of the staff using the machine carelessly will be quickly rebuked and if it is put in a cupboard and only used to do a fraction of the blood counts, there is a very critical enquiry by the manager or director. However, expenditure on equipment accounts for only some 10 per cent of the total annual cost. Yet how are staff treated? Any difficult technician tends to be pushed into a backwater and labelled as having a personality problem. Often technicians showing above-average ability and enthusiasm are left in jobs well below their capacity. Again, senior staff may never be instructed in the supervision or selection of staff. Frequently no attempt is made to assess staff performance as technicians are paid on a national scale whether they work hard or not and whether they keep up to date or not. There is a strong case for attempting to understand how staff behave and why in the interests of efficiency. But there is a much stronger one in terms of liberating the enthusiasm, creativity and drive which all staff possess regardless of professional group. These ideas are not intended to be a complete picture of present thinking by industrial psychologists and sociologists but are intended only to highlight ideas of particular relevance; to provide a few signposts as a guide to an alternative point of view; and to encourage further study. The following ideas are drawn from current views of such people as Professor T. Lupton, H. Schein, Professor Sprott, Munro Fraser and J. A. C. Brown (Lupton, 1966; Schein, 1965; Sprott, 1958; Fraser, 1965; Brown, 1954).

DEVELOPMENT OF PERSONALITY

A baby is born into a situation in which it is completely dependent on its parents for such needs as food, warmth and clothing. It is its early experience of how, through a dependent relationship, these need are satisfied, that forms the basis of the central or core personality. Early experience of success or failure with trial and error methods will determine whether a child feels secure or insecure first with its parents and later with its teacher and finally, in adult life, with the boss. Habits are established by some sort of reward and punishment system. Those habits and techniques which have been found to be effective by trial and error are built into the personality. Broadly speaking a child whose needs have been readily satisfied in this dependency situation will have strong social needs and a child whose needs have not been satisfied will have strong ego needs. Since no parent is completely satisfying or completely frustrating the child will have a mixture of social and ego needs. The balance between them—depending initially on the parents—is developed later by the teacher and other children.

During the first five years a child is learning not only how to control eating and excretion; it also learns how to deal with people, realizing that the best way to gain attention is by smiling or being naughty—particularly if it feels it is not getting enough attention. If by retiring into his shell or by pretending to be sick or hurt he finds he keeps out of trouble, these techniques or attitudes become part of the central or core personality because they have been successful. Since the individual personality comprises an integrated set of responses to life as he has experienced it, he feels a strong need to maintain it rigidly at all costs and will resist efforts to change it. This core personality may be modified by later experience though never entirely obliterated.

On the other hand the superficial or peripheral personality comes from the experience of an adult in society generally and particularly at work and is therefore influenced by accepted standards of behaviour and attitudes at work. Sociologists believe that a great deal of human behaviour which is supposed to come from a fixed characteristic is in fact a function of the individual in a group of people. A man's behaviour at work will be quite different from his behaviour at home with his family. Many chief technicians don this peripheral personality when they put on their white coat each morning. People generally tend to form a rigid picture of others simply because they see them only in one or two settings; for example, technicians seeing their boss as a tyrant would be astonished to see him relaxing at home pruning his roses. Similarly a chief technician who is tough with his technicians may be acquiescent with consultants. It is the same man in each case but he is using techniques which he feels appropriate to each situation, for though toughness may be successful with technicians, it will not work with consultants.

Generally speaking core personality is rigid and difficult to change while peripheral personality is more easily changed, particularly by current experience. It is common to hear a difficult technician described as having a personality problem and because it is accepted that human nature cannot be changed no further effort is made. This assumption is only true as far as core personality goes; it is not true of peripheral personality. One possible solution is to try changing the person's experience.

Human Needs

Humans have a range of needs which can be arranged in three major groups. The first is the need for food, warmth and shelter because without this the individual would not survive. The second need is for the company of other humans—that is a social need. Man feels lonely and deprived without the company of others and

118

this basic need in one human personality makes itself felt quite as insistently, though not in such obvious and understandable forms, as the need for food and warmth. The third major need is for status (ego need) or the need to be esteemed, recognized, well regarded or cared about. Some industrial psychologists add two more groups but though each person wants to be taken notice of and to have some sort of impact on other people some consider these to be subsections of ego needs. There is the need for autonomy—for man to know that he has some control over his destiny and that he is still the captain of his soul. Finally man has a need to use all his skills and resources and a need to feel he is doing a good job—this is described as self-actualization.

Each person has this range of needs and in a particular order of priority. As one need is met so the next in order of priority becomes the most urgent and as a need is satisfied so it loses its motivational force. The need for food, warmth and clothing is not a strong motivational force in laboratory staff nor is the need to be with a group of people as this is a normal everyday occurrence. So next in the order of priorities for most people are ego needs and these motivate much of the behaviour in pathology departments today. Many arguments about promotion are not really about money, the sum involved is often quite small, but about recognition and the need to 'be someone'. Senior staff are dropping out of the 'on-call' rota, in spite of the high income which can be earned, because of the low esteem in which 'on-call' staff are held, in that they are expected to behave mechanically.

Individual priorities of needs are not fixed and change depending on circumstances. A man getting what he considers is a reasonable share of attention is reasonably happy but if he feels he is overlooked, disregarded or taken for granted then he reacts at once. A great deal of the minor unpleasantness in everyday life is due to bruised ego. Ego satisfaction is a basic human need.

HUMAN NEEDS AND THEIR SATISFACTION

The social and ego needs of man are satisfied by belonging to groups of one sort and another, mostly at work. If a strong need is unsatisfied it gives rise to considerable tension and drive. Need satisfaction as an aspect of human personality is difficult to explain but it is most important in understanding human behaviour.

The problem facing each human is to find an outlet for his drive and to satisfy his need among the opportunities presented by his particular way of life. If he has a range of satisfying activities in work and leisure he will be happy and fulfilled but if he fails to find outlets in the normal range of activities available to him then his essential energy will be dammed up and will eventually drain away into disguised and perhaps destructive and antisocial outlets. If he cannot find satisfaction for his ego needs at work, he may pour his energy into his professional body or trade union where he will be accepted as someone having status. A student may seem lazy and unco-operative in the laboratory yet be prepared to train a couple of nights a week and play football every Saturday afternoon thus finding social satisfaction which his job is failing to provide for him. Senior staff with a dull monotonous job may look forward to 'on-call' duties if they can provide more satisfaction. So it is only when the job itself presents, or seems by the individual to present, opportunities for self-actualization and satisfaction of ego and social needs that he will be interested in co-operating to promote efficiency. Manipulation by monetary rewards alone cannot compensate for the absence of other satisfactions. Instances of this can be seen at once by anyone who looks at the jobs of his subordinates and their reactions to them.

Brown (1954) states that work is an essential part of a man's life since it is that aspect of his life which gives him status and binds him to society. When a man does not like work, the fault lies in the psychological and social conditions of the job. Work is a social activity. The morale of workers has no direct relationship whatsoever with the material conditions of the job, and of the many motives which make a man work, under normal conditions, money is one of the least important.

HUMAN BEHAVIOUR

There are many assumptions about human behaviour which do not fit observable facts but there are two basic ideas which are widely accepted by psychologists. First, all human behaviour is caused, it requires a stimulus and does not just happen spontaneously. Secondly it has a goal or a purpose, although this may not be recognized. These ideas can be presented diagrammatically.

Stimulus———→A Need or Want———→Goal

A need or want gives rise to tension and discomfort until it is satisfied. Reaching the goal satisfies the need and inactivates it as a motive. Human behaviour can largely be explained by reference to satisfaction or frustration of human needs as described earlier. The particular method of satisfying them will be determined by a person's background and their particular reference group.

Perception

Behaviour is how people set about satisfying their needs as they perceive them and this involves the idea of perception. Many people realize that the world is not exactly what it appears to be and that what is heard may not always be what is said because people tend to see what they want to see or hear what they want to hear. Perception is influenced by both needs and fears. A hungry man will look at food being offered by a pretty girl and not at the girl, but a man who has just eaten will not bother with the food. To ignore perception is to ignore a major determinant of human behaviour. It is the world as it is perceived which is important as far as human behaviour is concerned.

Thus a senior technician, seeking promotion to chief technician, will appreciate the status of the higher grade rather than the extra pay. So a manager must try to discover first of all the personal views of people and what they regard as fact. If he is to change their behaviour and if that behaviour is largely determined by their perception of the environment, then it is critical to understand the circumstances under which behaviour could change.

Response to Frustration

Inability to reach a goal leads to frustration and reaction to this may be directed either to the cause of the frustration or to a scapegoat in place of the real cause. Reaction may also be shame at an inability to cope with frustration or to rationalize the cause. Broadly speaking if a person is optimistic about his ability he will see the obstacle and his anger will be directed towards it. If, on the other hand, he is pessimistic about his ability his anger will be directed against himself. Many obstacles are depriving rather than frustrating because the obstacle does not seem insurmountable or the goal is not important to the person. Some people may therefore meet few frustrations because they perceive more ways round an obstacle or because they know their self-esteem does not have to be proved afresh by every problem which they encounter. Serious frustration may lead to specific types of behaviour which have been classified into four groups by Maier (1961). He distinguishes aggression, regression, resignation and fixation.

Aggression

Aggression may be the normal response of a busy person to frustration but it may also appear as a fight over every unimportant detail of a problem—such as bullying the junior nurse who brings the wrong specimen to a pathology department.

Regression

This can be recognized in childish behaviour, whispering in cliques and in a yearning for the good old days which were not always so good and in any case can never return. It can be heard echoing in the comment 'students would never have behaved like this in my day'.

Resignation

A failure to respond at all characterizes resignation, of which the following are instances: 'Thank goodness I have only a few more years to go before retiring'; 'Why bother to make an effort, things will never change'; 'It is not worth the effort they never listen'.

Fixation

Less common and more serious than the first three, fixation is compulsive or repetitive behaviour not directed towards a goal. Fixation also shows in the attitudes of those who resist change or persist in outdated and ineffective methods. The difficulty with people exhibiting this type of behaviour is that they are not amenable to rational argument or persuasion or even responsive to punishment.

Within pathology departments frustration shows up in any of the following ways: increased absenteeism, increased sickness rate, staff leaving, high accident rate and low rates of work, and industrial diseases such as dermatitis.

Conflict

Human behaviour has been described as goal-orientated or purposeful but life is rarely so simple. Conflict can arise when there is a choice of equally appealing goals; as when a women wants to continue her career in medical technology but also to get married and raise a family. Again it may be a senior technician who wants to be popular with his staff and yet run an efficient department. Much apparent laziness is probably the result of goal conflict in people; when the goals are equally pleasant or unpleasant no move is made in either direction. Tension and conflict **are** always much sharper when someone's core personality is being challenged or shown to be unpleasant or weak. The tension rises very quickly as it becomes necessary to revise a man's self-image for he will go to great lengths to preserve this.

Conflict often results from the need to belong to a group and yet be independent as in adolescence. Again a weak chief technician working for a more forceful pathologist may feel conflict between being protected by the strong superior and yet losing autonomy in the process.

Much supervision at work is really an attempt to control staff through the use of conflict, because threats of discipline to prevent or obtain certain behaviour is only an attempt to introduce conflict into another person's conceptual world.

Active conflict may show itself as anxiety, unpredictable lashing-out against subordinates, inexplicable refusal to delegate authority, and self-isolation from peers and, if possible, from superiors.

People learn to live together to satisfy their human needs but at the same time must accept some restriction. Although conflict between individuals and their social environment is always present, it can be accepted and regarded as reasonable. When this happens a well adjusted member of society will result, in that he follows the behaviour which the society considers normal. If restrictions are not accepted he will be in conflict with his social environment. However, where situations are changing rapidly an individual may find it more difficult to adapt satisfactorily to the norms of the group to which he belongs—as with post-war technicians and the I.M.L.T.

Human Behaviour at Work

The psychology of the individual as described by Jung or Freud is not very helpful in trying to understand the behaviour of people at work. It is relatively recently, in the last 15 years, that sociologists have pointed out how the individual can never be understood by himself but must always be viewed in relation to the group in which he is situated at the time when his behaviour is being considered. A manager who hopes to understand the behaviour of a subordinate and more important his own behaviour, must understand the structure and characteristics of primary and secondary groups first of all.

GROUPS

Primary groups are small informal groups within which people are in face-to-face relationships with each other, as in a laboratory, and large secondary or formal groups are those in which relationships have to be more contractual, such as in a pathology department. For a detailed discussion readers are referred to the authors listed at the end of the book (Sprott, 1958; Brown, 1954).

This chapter is mainly concerned with informal primary groups at work and the effect of them on the individual and the organization, and only to a lesser extent with secondary groups. (Secondary groups are discussed briefly first therefore.) It is also concerned with the way in which people's behaviour changes as they move from one group to another and what influence the primary group has on their attitudes and behaviour.

Secondary Groups

These groups are larger ones formed to carry out a job; such as a hospital's staff or pathology department staff. Only certain specified activities are carried out and the staff are given ranks and formed into some sort of hierarchy in which they are expected to behave according to their rank and carry out their formal duties in an impersonal and stereotyped way.

Primary Groups

Man has needs beyond the minimum needs of doing his job and will seek to satisfy them by developing a series of relationships with other staff. So whenever from 4–12 people come together, particularly if they already have similar jobs or status because of work or physical proximity, they will tend to form a group which will then assign to its members roles and status. The more people interact the more they like each other and are at ease in each other's company, tending to develop a common understanding and language.

Group culture

A primary group will develop some form of organization which defines status, depending on the contribution a person makes to the group, and the function of each member. One may be the organizer, one the clown (butt for any joke), another the group's conscience and another the accepted leader. The group also tends to prescribe attitudes to those in and those outside the group. It will also require of its members some conformity of behaviour and aspirations. These standards of behaviour or group norms will set the tempo and determine the characteristics of the group. They help to identify and define it and thereby to establish the status of the individual. Acceptance of group norms promotes group goals because it facilitates the establishment of working procedures, co-ordination and the discipline of individual contributions. Group norms are shared by members because of the potential sanctions the group can invoke in the case of deviants. The application of pressure to conform can take a wide variety of forms from sending a member to Coventry, or withholding information, to excluding him from informal and formal social functions.

The relationship of the individual to the group will vary from fully conforming to non-conforming when the person will physically be a member but in effect totally isolated within the group. Some may be members of a particular group but accept their standards from another group which they consider to be more important or from their reference group: for example, a pathologist may be a member of a primary group of laboratory staff but then take his standards and group norms from the hospital consultants who are his reference group. In the same way the biochemist may take his group norms from outside the pathology department.

Each group will tend to create some sort of mechanism to check member's behaviour and may even bring sanctions to bear if necessary. These matters are a part of the group relationships and not something that is added on or imposed. Members find a balance between the advantages of co-operating and accepting group norms and those of going outside them.

Finally a satisfactory group will be one which offers its members a status high enough to be satisfactory (having regard to his personality), a role wide enough and a satisfactory degree of security in this role and status based on mutual understanding.

Group Function for the Individual

The main function of a group for individual members is to satisfy their social needs but it does more than this. It provides support for members and an opportunity to practise behaviour and skills. It gives each member a sense of identity and a measure of self-esteem. Through group membership a person can develop or confirm some feeling of identity again and thereby enhance his self-esteem. Status, if only as the clown of the group, is better than nothing.

The group provides an opportunity for a member to establish and test reality; to have his view confirmed that the chief technician is a slave driver for example or that a houseman is sending in ridiculous requests. Uncertain parts of the social environment can

125

be made real and stable by checking out with other group members.

Group membership provides increased security for individual members and increases their power to cope with a common powerful enemy or threat. Technicians in a laboratory will feel more secure in standing up to the hospital secretary for example as a group than as individuals.

Groups provide a way of ensuring co-operation to get work done and activity to fill any leisure time at work. Thus, a group may play cards together during the lunch hour or eat at the same table in the dining-room.

In establishing a set of group norms the primary group is the instrument of society through which, in large measure, the individual acquires his attitudes and opinions, goals and ideas. It is also one of the fundamental sources of discipline and this is generally a much stronger discipline than that imposed by the boss.

Effect of the Group on Individuals

Status in the formal or secondary group is derived from a person's rank, thus a pathologist has a higher status than a chief technician. In the primary group status is related to skill, not just skill at work but any skill the group finds useful, such as organizing social functions, however small, or helping members who are in any sort of trouble, or perhaps skill in getting the boss to agree to a particular course of action which the members want. Members tend to stimulate each other and most people are more productive when working in a group than by themselves. Once a group norm has been formed members' judgments, even in private, tend to be the same. It is understandable therefore that it is more difficult to change the views of a single member than the views of the group as a whole. A change brought about in group norm or attitude will be more permanent and more likely to be accepted if all members participate in the discussion. The minority in the group tend to move to the views of the majority.

Group Function for the Organization

The group works both for and against the organization. A primary group usually insists that members do a fair day's work and it may also help to get work done by side-stepping the formal organization. If a senior technician is a friend of the electrician he probably gets electrical equipment repaired more quickly than he could by using the formal channels. The primary group also gives members an opportunity to step out of their position in the

126

formal organization by dropping in on another group member for a cup of tea and a cigarette.

The primary group, as has already been said, has a powerful influence on its members' behaviour and can undermine the authority of the boss and prevent his orders being carried out effectively particularly if they seem to oppose the group norms. A primary group can slow the work down if it feels it is being subject to pressure or attack in any way. Just as an individual's behaviour can only be understood in relation to the group in which he is functioning, so the behaviour of the group can only be understood in the context of the larger group to which it belongs.

Group Leaders

The group will select leaders who provide the best skill to meet any particular job to be done. If the task is negotiating with the hospital secretary for use of the hospital tennis court the group may not necessarily choose the chief technician but the person who is most likely to succeed with the job. Yet another person may be chosen to organize the Christmas party because he has a flair for doing this. In the event of a threatened strike the group will choose the militant man who under normal circumstances would be disregarded.

The way in which a group performs is dependent in many ways on the leader's style or method of leading. Experiments have shown that a democratic leadership gives rise to more personal and friendly relationships. More individual differences were shown among members and yet at the same time members were more group minded and looked to one another for mutual approval. There was less scapegoating and a steadier level of work even in the absence of the leader. Ineffective or *laissez-faire* leadership created a less effective group in terms of work; members asked many more questions and work decreased when the leader was absent. Finally an authoritarian style of leadership provoked two patterns of behaviour. The group were either aggressive or apathetic and in each case showed a strong dependence on the leader. The aggressive reaction involved a rebelliousness and a demanding of attention from the leader. Groups found it very difficult to respond to dramatic changes in the style of leadership.

It has been found that supervisors of high-production groups were under less supervision from their own boss and placed less direct emphasis upon production as a goal. They encouraged employees to participate in making decisions and were more concerned with their staff than with the work. They spent more time in supervision and less time in straight productive work. The supervisors had a greater feeling of confidence in their own supervisory work and felt they knew where they stood with the company. These findings on group leadership have obvious implications for director, manager and technologist in pathology departments.

It is not being suggested that any one should alter their style of leadership to one which is foreign to their nature. The effects would be obvious and distasteful to their subordinates. What is essential is that it be recognized that a manager's style has pronounced effects on the behaviour of his subordinates. If a manager is tough and authoritarian by nature then he must learn to live with the results rather than to blame his subordinates for their behaviour.

The major problem for a manager is to balance the needs of the organization with the needs of primary groups in his department. A successful manager is one who persuades primary groups to accept any goals which he regards as desirable as their own.

Effects of Communication Patterns

Good communications are commonly said to be vital to good relationships and it is often felt that the communications cannot be good where organization is not clearly defined. As every one at work spends a lot of time giving and receiving information, ideas and instruction, it follows that information should be accurate and relevant. Orders and instruction should be clear and unambiguous and people should be clear what they have to do and have the necessary information to carry out the job. If communications are one-way and people are simply told what to do without a chance to ask questions or check on detail, there is a greater chance of a mistake. If people are given an opportunity to understand the reason for the instruction and ask questions in order to clarify the instruction, however, they are more likely to co-operate. This supports the concept that good communications are closely linked with good organization and relationships.

However, recent experiments show that this relationship is not true. The communication system in a department may be considered as a network among staff and the communication pattern in a group will affect people's behaviour in such things as the activity and satisfaction of members, emergence of leaders and organization of the group, and the speed with which problems are solved.

In *Figure 7a* the chief technician will emerge as the leader giving information to and receiving information from all the senior technicians and so he will get much more satisfaction out of his job than the senior technicians who exchange information only with the chief technician. In *Figure 7b* in which everyone communicates with everyone else the chief technician is less likely to emerge as the leader, problems will not be solved as quickly, but everyone will get a great deal more satisfaction from the process. Experiments also show that the network outlined in *Figure 7b* is more adaptable to change in the type of situation or the type of information.

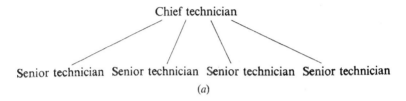

(*a*)

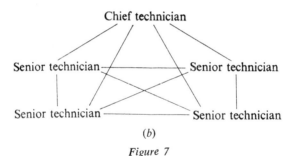

(*b*)

Figure 7

An efficient department is faced with a choice between two approaches. Speedy and direct communications for quickly solving problems but creating low satisfaction and morale among staff. (The short-run gain of rapid problem solving will here be offset by the decrease in morale.) And the alternative all round two-way communication, slower problem solving, and greater satisfaction on the part of the staff.

Two-way communication is said to be good and hence people will be satisfied. Experiments show that one-way communications are faster and more effective where routines are well established and speed of communication is important. Two-way communications are more effective if accuracy is important but they have the disadvantage that where the communicator is someone in authority it can show up mistakes and undermine confidence. An uncertain or insecure chief technician may use one-way communication to avoid his uncertainty or other shortcomings being exposed. Two-way communications can also be distorted by differences in rank: as for example, a pathologist giving instruction to a new student.

All this suggests that there is no straightforward relationship between good communications, efficiency and satisfaction. Up and down and side-way communications of clearly expressed information and ideas may increase satisfaction but might hinder speedy decisions and produce uncertainty, blurring of the message and other faults. One-way communications from a powerful person may make for a speedy and efficient working in the short run but produce dissatisfaction and long-run inefficiency.

Intergroup Conflict

Many people run their department by dividing and ruling their staff but there is now considerable evidence to suggest that intergroup conflict is bad in the long run. Competing groups tend to become more close-knit—more concerned with work than with members' needs. The leadership pattern becomes more autocratic and so the group becomes more highly structured, demanding high loyalty. Competing groups see each other as the enemy and can only hear or see the bad things in the other group. There is increasing hostility and decreasing interaction and communication between them. Any discussion between the two groups will only be concerned with finding fault with each other. Intergroup conflict may make each group more effective in the short run but the groups become far less satisfying to their members. The winning group becomes more tightly knit and shows release of tension, becoming more happy and showing a high degree of co-operation between members and increased concern for individual member's needs. The losing group look for a reason for their defeat claiming the judge was biased, or the rules were wrong and looking for a scapegoat in consequence. Again the losing group tends to splinter and any old feuds will flair up. There is low intergroup co-operation and less concern about individual member's needs. The negative consequences far outweigh the positive ones.

Problems and Large Organizations

As hospitals grow larger staff are members of increasingly large secondary groups which demand more formal or contractual behaviour than do primary groups and are less satisfying. The membership of several secondary groups can make demands on people which they find difficult to meet because there is confusion between professional standards and managerial expediency. A pathologist on the Medical Staff Committee and the Hospital Management Committee may find his professional views clashing with managerial reality. A chief technician as departmental manager will feel the conflict between his role as departmental manager and that of a technologist.

Effect of Organizational Changes on Primary Groups

The rotation of student technicians through all the various laboratories in pathology departments for training purposes has made it difficult for them to find a primary group and be accepted. This is reflected in the high wastage of students in very large pathology departments. Such rotation has made it increasingly difficult for technologists to weld their staff into a primary group as half of them stay for only six months.

The technologist gained his status in the working group from exclusive technical skill. He introduced and performed new techniques, and in the past kept them to himself for long periods. Today with the pressure of work and the speed of development in technology new techniques, using complex equipment, are introduced by the technologist and usually are rapidly passed on to the subordinates thus tending to reduce the status of technologists.

The transition from evening classes for technicians to block-release classes has come about in 4 or 5 years, which is a relatively short time when compared with the engineering students who took 20 years to make the same change. The effects of this rapid transition are only just being felt but no doubt will continue to be felt for the next 10 years.

Senior technicians resent junior students being given 10 weeks off each year and pathologists do not see the point of teaching students such a wide range of academic subjects. The heated correspondence in the Gazette I.M.L.T. concerning General Studies is a symptom of this sudden transition.

Automation has brought with it strong reactions from workers in many fields; for example, the coal industry, the docks and the motor car industry and there is reason to assume the same response will occur in pathology departments. The various symptoms arising from the introduction of automation have been well described

(Brown, 1954). Any person introducing automation in pathology departments should at least be aware of the response he is likely to provoke. Automation may be necessary on economic grounds but without some consideration for human needs and information regarding primary groups the gains may be less than the losses.

IMPLICATIONS FOR MANAGERS

A successful manager is one who ensures that the purpose of his department is achieved but that at the same time the staff are able to satisfy their human needs within the context of their jobs. A manager whose open commitment to these two objectives is as obvious to his subordinates as this will act as a powerful motivator. His success in obtaining good results in both these objectives will also ensure the maximum effectiveness of his department. Given adequate technical skills in the managerial sense, a manager's strategy will depend on how well he understands people and their needs and how closely his assumptions about human needs and behaviour fit reality. The common assumptions about human needs and behaviour, which are in fact invalid, are summed up by McGregor (1960).

McGregor states that behind every management decision or action are assumptions about human nature and human behaviour and lists them as follows:

(1) The average human being has an inherent dislike of work and will avoid it if he can.

(2) Because of this human characteristic of dislike of work, most people must be coerced, controlled, directed and threatened with punishment to get them to put forth adequate effort towards the achievement of organizational objectives.

McGregor describes these assumptions as theory X and states that they are common among managers, in spite of the fact that there are many readily observable phenomena in industry and elsewhere which are not consistent with this view of human nature. At one time or another pathologists and technicians will have heard these views expressed by their colleagues about their subordinates. McGregor has formulated a number of generalizations (theory Y) from a knowledge of human nature, which provide for managers more realistic assumptions about human behaviour. These are:

(1) The expenditure of physical and mental effort in work is as natural as in play or rest.

132

(2) External control and the threat of punishment are not the only means of bringing about effort towards organization objectives. Man will exercise self-direction and self-control in the service of objectives to which he is committed.

(3) Commitment to objectives is a function of the reward associated with their achievement. The most significant of such rewards for example, satisfaction of ego and self-actualization needs, can be direct products of effort directed to organizational objectives.

(4) The average human being learns under proper conditions not only to accept but to seek responsibility.

(5) The capacity to exercise a relatively high degree of imagination, ingenuity and creativity in the solution of organizational problems is widely, not narrowly, distributed in the population.

(6) Under the conditions of modern industrial life, the intellectual potentialities of the average human being are only partially utilized.

Many pathologists and chief technicians still assume that promotion and higher pay are the only genuine incentives—subscribing to theory X—to get people to stay in their job and work harder. A different point of view has been put forward by Herzberg (Herzberg, Mausner and Snyderman, 1959). He sees the matter in terms of groups of motivators; in the first group there are, he suggests, the satisfiers such as achievement, recognition for achievement, responsibility, advancement and self-development—though he found their presence satisfied everyone, their absence did not make many dissatisfied. The second group Herzberg describes as hygiene factors in that their absence did not actively promote good morale but avoided bad morale. An analogy may be drawn in preventive public health work which does not promote good health but avoids ill health. These hygiene factors are: company policy and administration, supervision, relationship with supervisor, work conditions, effect on personal life of relationship with equals, relationships with subordinates, status and security. These factors are related to the context of the job and not to the job itself. He found their presence made men dissatisfied but their absence did not make them feel satisfied.

Besides knowing how other people behave it is important that the individual considers his own motives and behaviour. Subordinates have very sharp perception about their superior's motives which may not be recognized by the superior himself. The present style of medical education has induced certain attitudes in consultant pathologists as previously mentioned in Chapter 2. Technicians in general have an urgent need for increased status which influences their behaviour in pathology departments. One of the problems facing pathologists today is that of seeing and complementing the relative status needs of managers, technologists and technicians and not blocking these status and prestige needs in order to emphasize their own.

The pursuit of efficiency by the introduction of automation and centralization which deprives staff as individuals and as groups of satisfaction is commonplace in pathology departments; in recent years to some extent this dissatisfaction is compensated for by higher grades and pay but many staff, chief technicians in particular, are seeking satisfaction outside their work: for example, by writing books, actively supporting their professional bodies and trade unions and by teaching. There is no support for the idea that human needs must be satisfied in order to obtain an efficient department in the short run. The evidence is that the effects of frustration caused by the pursuit of efficiency are part of the price of efficiency.

High staff turnover, absenteeism, increased time lost through sickness and the like are forms of adaptive behaviour, and must be considered as symptoms and a search made for the cause. Managers require a diagnostic approach in order to minimize them and a careful study of pathology departments, jobs and relationships within pathology departments.

Essentially, the manager has to find ways of pursuing efficiency which within the limits imposed by financial and technological factors, will do the least damage to individuals.

CHAPTER 8

FUTURE SCIENTIFIC SERVICES IN THE N.H.S.

INTRODUCTION

The reader may well ask why he should attempt to put into operation the ideas covered in the previous chapters. There are good reasons, for most senior staff feel they have not sufficient time to seriously consider tomorrow's problems and this is a symptom of their inability to cope satisfactorily with today's work as it takes up all their time and energy. Most of them feel vaguely dissatisfied with the way in which they are doing their work, crash programmes seem all to frequently to be called for and in spite of them the same problems tend to recur. Judging from the comments of the three professional bodies it is apparent that their members are uncertain about their future.

Generally speaking the demand for information from clinicians seems to be expanding faster than the available money and staff. As work in each laboratory increases so the pathologist becomes more dependent on technicians for greater effort, enthusiasm and skill and these will be needed even more in future. Unfortunately the present relationship and attitudes between the three groups are not likely to produce this co-operation. Even if technicians found answers to some of the difficulties they would be unlikely to suggest them to a pathologist who was indifferent to their needs as individuals. The best way to encourage technicians to work harder is to accept them as full members of the team in a pathology department in which their personal and social needs are considered.

It is sometimes argued that problems are made worse because the H.M.C. has its financial priorities wrong; the Regional Board does not understand; the Ministry of Health is out of touch; or the wrong political party is in power. These arguments, whether true or not, are often used as an excuse to avoid examining personal efficiency and tackling problems within departments. Although it is difficult, pathologists, biochemists and technicians need to stand back from their work and ask themselves what is the purpose of their department and if they are making the best use of their resources to achieve this purpose.

It would be wrong to suggest that pathology departments in this country are not good: indeed, they are the envy of many other countries. Until now they have been allowed to evolve without much planning but the great changes taking place in hospitals and in medical practice mean that this evolutionary system is too slow and uncertain. Over the past 20 years pathologists, biochemists and technicians have been able to develop new skills with changes but the rate is now too fast to allow this. Bagrit discussing computers in his Reith Lectures (1966), said that in future everyone will have to be retrained at least once in his working life. This is true of pathology staff today because the various jobs are different today from what they were 10 years ago and this difference must become greater each year. Thus some sort of retraining will be required by the three groups of staff in the next few years.

Many of the solutions being put forward to problems arising in pathology departments today make assumptions which are not supported by current experience. A common theme is regionalization or centralization and yet there are few, if any, successful examples of co-operation on a regional or subregional basis. Regional Pathology Advisory Committees have chosen not to provide strong and clear leadership in obtaining co-operation between pathology departments. Attempts to organize technicians' training on a subregional basis have failed. Even co-operation between pathology departments in the same H.M.C. can amount to little more than an armed truce. Some attempts will have to be made to understand the causes of this and to look for solutions at H.M.C. level before any scheme for organizing pathology on a regional basis has a chance of succeeding.

Pathology staff do not see their job as anything other than medical or scientific and feel that other work, for example, management and administration is something to be done only when their professional and technical work is finished. They should be helped to appreciate that the effectiveness and efficiency of their department is largely dependent on their skill as directors, managers and technologists.

The problems which have been discussed in this book are not peculiar to pathology departments; they exist in scientific establishments in industry, with the same difficulties arising in solving problems. The following passage, taken from 'Human Problems of Innovation' (Problems in Industry No. 5 H.M.S.O., 1967) illustrates the point admirably:

136

In the presence of rapid technical change and the strain it imposes, two natural human reactions can be recognized, and with vigour and steadiness, guarded against and countered. One is the impulse to scurry back for safety to the mechanical system, the authority of the chief and the book of rules. It is totally inappropriate. The other is to blame the personal defects and shortcomings of the individuals concerned. Whether or not they contribute to the trouble, it has deeper causes.

These are negative prescriptions. Positive prescriptions must obviously be differently interpreted in every firm according to the nature of its task, the abilities of the staff and the starting point of the structure. The first and most constant requirement is that management should constantly re-examine what the firm is supposed to be doing, with the conscious aim of adopting operating methods and the structure of managerial relationships to its present task. There is no question of any particular structure being better or worse than another; everything depends on circumstances. If the task of the firm can in fact be carried out by a number of people each with a specific set of responsibilities and correspondingly limited liabilities, each occupying a well established place in a pyramid of authority, so much the better; such a system in the right circumstances, is economical and effective and has the great advantage of imposing far less wear and tear stress and uncertainty, on individuals. But when the firm is tackling new tasks, commercial or technical, this system of differentiated routine functions will not do. Delimitations must be made fluid, responsibilities must be elastically shared. Every effort must be made to encourage the sense of the business as a whole, with objectives and goals common to all its members rather than a complex of separate jobs. The stronger this sense, the more recourse to lateral consultation which should be recognized and facilitated, not regarded as mere semi-legitimate supplement to the vertical channels of command.

Putting these prescriptions into effect is partly a matter of organization, as in the example cited above, of recasting of the productive structure into development teams. Partly, also, it is a more difficult matter of tone and style; of establishing as the done and recognized thing, a code of mutual good manners expressing—at whatever level of formality or informality—a spirit of co-operation and appreciation rather than a desire to score or assert prestige. The firm should in fact regard the continuous deliberate recasting of its own structure, the establishment of organic relationships, and the maintenance of a social climate in which these can flourish as no less important a part of the innovating process than the building of laboratories and the recruitment of scientists and technologists.

In attempting to cure some of the ills prevalent in pathology departments, an accurate diagnosis will have to precede treatment for there is no single cure and no single way of managing a department successfully. Revans (1964) noted that: 'Hospitals need to start learning to understand themselves better and this learning process can only take place when it is tackled voluntarily by those on the spot'. A diagnostic approach is necessary because pathologists and chief technicians have only a vague idea of the non-technical content of their own or their subordinates' jobs. It will vary between laboratories, making it impossible to write a single job description. Any attempt to cure problems before a detailed analysis of the situation has been made will fail or at best only be partially successful. Pathologists, biochemists and technicians need to meet on neutral ground, in an unemotional atmosphere and try to identify problems and causes of conflict. This would not work so well at national level where people tend to be steeped in the ambitions and politics of professional bodies.

This book has attempted to describe the activities of the pathology department of a District General Hospital and hence is based on a common denominator but in practice many such departments may be different. It has also attempted to define the purpose of the department and criteria for effectiveness and efficient performance, together with some techniques and ideas which are helpful. It can, however, only direct the attention of the top team to problems in their own department. No one learns from reading theories from a book as learning can only be made effective if facts are collected, examined and seen in a new light and, too, by trying out new ideas and new attitudes. Education is a continuous process and cannot be achieved in a crash course; it must also be interdisciplinary and interprofessional.

The first step in management training should be to encourage staff to take a wider view of their department and its activities and to see that planning, co-ordinating, measuring performance and educating are essential activities. The second step comes from the staff when they decide they need extra skills to do their job to their satisfaction. The personal identification of specific training requirements is important, as successful learning is more likely when the learner is well motivated.

Two very important results will stem from the application of the ideas in the previous chapters. Firstly, the fuller understanding of all staff's activities—scientific, managerial and supervisory—will mean fewer crash programmes will be needed to solve difficulties and staff will find that they are becoming more effective but with less effort. Secondly with this approach they will save time; in this they will be able to anticipate some of tomorrow's problems.

TOMORROW

So far the discussion has been about today's problems but what about tomorrow? To begin with it is essential to assess the future needs of clinicians and the sort of pathology service they will want from pathology departments. This means looking for the indications or trends in their present activities.

The structure of the N.H.S. is likely to undergo major changes within the next few years. The one idea common to all suggestions is the integration of the three sections of the N.H.S.—the hospital service, the general practitioners and the services provided by local authorities. Stevens (1966) sees three broad trends: (a) the changing role of the general practitioner with his need to work more closely with hospitals and specialists and the requirement for a new kind of generalism; (b) the central position of the hospital in providing specialist services and thus increasingly all kinds of medical services; and finally (c) the development of professional organizations to control the standards of post-graduate education, which has now become the period of practical specialized training. It may therefore be assumed that the pathology departments will become both less orientated towards hospital clinicians and more concerned with a wider range of clinicians with differing needs. As more money becomes available, the medical officer of health or whoever takes his place, will use pathology departments to provide facilities for population screening. The limited experience of the exfoliative cytology screening suggests that not enough is known about the most effective economical way of organizing such a service.

As general practitioners move into group practice, as seems likely, and become more closely associated with hospitals, they will no doubt make greater use of the scientific services. Hospitals' beds will be used more for treatment than for diagnosis as at present. This trend would mean more tests on out-patients. Medical practice now includes intensive-care units which call for continuous monitoring of patients and pathology departments will be expected to provide increasing amounts of simple information much more rapidly than at present. This poses new problems regarding the collection of specimens and the rapid return of information. Only a few investigations into this sort of problem have been published so far.

Most of the necessary technical knowledge is available to provide a large number of tests, or multiple screening at low cost per test but until doctors are ready to cope with these, its introduction will have to wait. New economical methods must be designed for handling and analysing the significant facts which emerge from the mass of information that could be provided. In spite of the low cost per test the total expenditure for multiple screening is very high in relation to the amount of money available through the N.H.S. As yet there is no evidence to support the view that more money spent on pathology departments, enabling them to provide a bigger and faster service, will shorten the length of patients' stay in hospital. Until doctors are able to make full use of the information provided in pathology reports at present there is no point in extending the service.

Many difficulties experienced by pathology departments today stem from the faulty organization of clinical teams. These difficulties will diminish if the report of the joint Working Party on the Organization of Medical Work in Hospitals (1967) is put into practice. They recommend that specialities should be grouped into divisions under a chairman and that one of their functions should be to consider the use of resources, for both medical ancillary services and equipment and so work out the optimum usage. This would involve liaison with other divisions and with non-medical groups.

The N.H.S. planners are envisaging changes in the structure and organization of future hospitals. The spate of Reports of various committees, Salmon (1966), Hunt (1966), Cogwheel (1967), Zuckerman (1968), H.M. 28 (68) Ministry of Health (1968b) and the Green Paper of July 1968 Ministry of Health (1968a) set out the framework of the N.H.S. at national, regional and hospital level. They do not suggest cures for existing problems but propose a framework within which people can create an effective and efficient service if they want to. Whatever the final outcome, pathology departments have to assess the new situation and adopt new and appropriate strategies particularly in relation to the proposed Area Health Boards. Planners are talking of grouping all services, including pathology, at one industrial site in a given area. They are designing new systems for handling information and two hospitals have recently installed computers to handle all internal information including pathology reports. It is clear that in future pathology departments will have to arrange their methods of handling reports to fit in with such systems. The speed and complexity of treatment will render the delivery of reports by hand obsolete in a few years' time, though the shortage of money may force the retention of this system until electronic systems become cheaper.

Future Resources

In the past most equipment used in pathology departments has either been built or designed in the U.S.A. or has been adapted from industrial equipment in this country. The system of each department purchasing its own equipment has prevented the N.H.S. influencing manufacturers as a large customer would normally do. Neither the Central Pathology Advisory Committee nor the Technicians' Consultative Committee have been able to alter this situation and until the last few years professional bodies have not been interested in the design of scientific equipment. The Ministry of Health set up in 1966 a group to investigate the development of screening techniques using automatic equipment linked to data processing systems with computerized recording calculation and control. Another group has been formed to advise on the development and testing of new laboratory equipment. They are working in close association with the Supplies Division of the Ministry of Health, with the scientific instrument industry and with the group investigating automatic equipment. It is to be hoped that both groups include someone with a knowledge of ergonomics and that an industrial psychologist or sociologist is looking at the possible ill effects of automation on staff as this may well be considerable and must be anticipated and forestalled as far as possible. The future of small pathology departments requires consideration if they are not to degenerate into sorting centres, doing only the simplest work themselves and sending the rest to a central department.

Staff

The majority of senior staff in pathology departments are in their early forties and will not be retiring for 20 years, so for this period they will continue to be the top team. People following on will be little better trained perhaps but, though basically the same, they will be expected to learn more rapidly and have a wider variety of skills. New staff will be more difficult to recruit because of greater competition among employers and the increased tendency to undertake further education after leaving secondary schools. They will require a new style of supervision because of their attitudes to authority and their social expectations. Training will be in greater depth but unless there is a change it will not provide all the skills that future staff will need such as in managing, supervising and organizing work. Staff will also tend to be promoted at an earlier age than at present, giving them less time and opportunity to learn by experience.

In order to keep pace with increasing work-loads the number of technicians employed in the N.H.S. needs to increase at the rate of 500 per year. While this was achieved in 1966 and 1967 prospects for maintaining it in future are only fair. For biochemists to keep pace with the increase in work they should increase at the rate of 25 per year whereas they have had an average increase of 17 per annum for the last ten years. Consultant pathologists should increase by 65 per annum but there is little hope of them doing so in the present medical manpower situation. The general conclusion is that the recruitment of all groups must be increased not only by improving career prospects but also by improving methods of recruitment.

Money

The Chief Medical Officer of the M.O.H. noted that money for the N.H.S. was not cut during the financial crisis of 1967 and 1968, but to provide a better service, money must be found out of the present allocation. This provides a difficult managerial task for directors and managers of pathology departments.

The financial position is not likely to improve within the next few years for hospitals and this will inevitably slow down the expansion of pathology departments. The average hospital financial allocation is increasing by about 1 per cent per annum while the expenditure of pathology departments is increasing by well over 10 per cent per annum and will have to taper off. Money for improvements and expansion will have to be found—mainly from the existing annual allocation of money—by improved efficiency and effectiveness. When eventually money becomes more readily available there will be fierce competition among all hospital departments for a bigger slice of the annual allocation but hospital administrators will be able to measure the efficiency of a department more easily and accurately so that departmental income will be more closely related to work-loads and efficiency than at present.

In spite of the substantial hospital building programme many pathology departments will be in old buildings well into the 1970s and some, in new buildings, will find themselves cramped for space. The hospital building notes have laid down standards but have not contributed to design and to date no single outstanding design has emerged.

THE ZUCKERMAN REPORT

So far the future needs of clinicians and future resources have been discussed; now it is necessary to consider what is the most suitable organization to provide the services required within the limits of available resources.

By 1966 the situation in the diagnostic departments had become serious. The effects of fragmentation of the service were obvious. In spite of heavy investment in automated equipment in pathology departments the national figures showed no increase in productivity—that is, in the number of tests per technician per annum; indeed this was beginning to decline. The lack of manpower planning was highlighted by the introduction of the National Certificate system for medical laboratory technicians. The distribution of courses through the country did not coincide with the wishes of pathology departments nor was any consideration given to the number of technicians that would be required with the H.N.C. qualification in Medical Laboratory Sciences. The growing shortage of medical manpower threw doubt on the value of the large number of consultant pathologists, constituting as they do some 12 per cent of all consultants in the N.H.S. There were no signs of the various professional bodies changing their views and attitudes and co-operating to consider the future of the scientific services. Against this background the Zuckerman Committee was set up: 'To consider the future organization and development of Hospital Scientific and Technical Services in the National Health Service hospitals and the broad pattern of staffing required and to make recommendations'.

Only a few bodies published their evidence before submitting it to the Zuckerman Committee. The evidence of the Association of Clinical Pathologists and the Association of Clinical Biochemists is too long to discuss in detail though it is worth reading. Their evidence emphasizes the difference in approach of the two groups and the way in which they see the proposed service in terms of pathologists and biochemists. The A.C.P. evidence seems to assume that pathology will not change much apart from needing a flexible team of laboratory staff. The change of duties of a chief technician is acknowledged by altering his title to that of laboratory supervisor but no comment is made on the changing and difficult relationship between chief technician and pathologist. Their complaints about national maldistribution of personnel and equipment suggests either that the Central and Regional Pathology Advisory Committees are not doing their job or that their terms of reference are wrong. Their complaints of local financial allocation being spasmodic, and of competition with other hospital departments puts responsibility on to each H.M.C. but, at the same time, ignores pathologists' lack of success at managing their departments. The fact that the A.C.P. offers no solution to these two difficulties, other than asking for special consideration, supports the view that they do not appreciate the need for managerial skills.

The evidence submitted by the I.M.L.T. Council seems to be a superficial and one-sided analysis, more concerned with technicians' career prospects than with the reorganization of the scientific and technical services in the N.H.S. The report suggests that existing problems in pathology departments arise from shortage of staff due to poor recruitment, training and career prospects and offers solutions only to technicians' problems making little comment on the organization of the service. The report is in keeping with the Institute Council's unspoken policy of not becoming involved in the running of the pathology service in hospitals and restricting their activities to what they feel are the 'best interests of their members'.

The A.C.B. report recommends a regional committee to control finance and staffing of all biochemistry laboratories in a region, presumably to side-track the present control by pathologists at hospital and regional level. This recommendation ignores the fact that pathology staff show little inclination to co-operate at local regional level at present. The formation of a regional committee does not automatically guarantee co-operation.

Pathologists and biochemists seem to be attempting in their evidence to solve problems by re-shaping the organization. This will not be successful as the problems are not primarily organizational: pathologists' difficulties stem, in the main, from their lack of managerial skill and biochemists' difficulties arise from changes in the triangular relationship of director, manager and technologist. Lasting improvement will only come from both recognition and a study of the above difficulties.

The general recommendations of the Zuckerman Report—the

unification of scientific services, regional and national chief scientists and the simplification of staff structure—are good and, in the main, were predictable. (An article initiated by A. P. Johnson entitled 'Laboratory Technicians' Evidence' and submitted by the Association of Scientific, Technical and Managerial Staff to the *British Hospital Journal and Social Service Review* of June 1968, was most timely in its appearance.) Some of the recommendations make a great deal of sense both in teaching hospitals and those attached to universities but rather less sense in medium and small district general hospitals. The general idea of a new division will sadden many administrators as they see their tripartite system likely to be replaced by a tetrapartite one. The proposed changes from the present democratic system to a relatively autocratic system of chief scientists will produce some interesting sociological symptoms but it is unlikely to lead to the flexible system hoped for.

In some ways the report is confirming reality in progressive district general hospitals. The chairman of the scientific services will, in the first instance, be a pathologist—a fact which will tend to draw him further away from the technical work. This is already happening as the total number of consultant pathologists is increasing less rapidly than the work for them and already there are unfilled vacancies for consultant pathologists in less favoured areas. The report envisages managerial jobs appearing but already a number of chief technicians are being accepted as departmental managers and acquiring managerial skills. Some technicians in pathology and medical physics departments, are being accepted as technologists and are introducing new ideas. The recommendation of a new grade for technical assistant is simply confirming the fact that junior technicians with O.N.C. or Intermediate I.M.L.T. examinations have been doing the bulk of the routine work for many years. The creation of a new grade of senior technical assistant will encourage this group to enlarge. Laboratory assistants or technical aides have already been introduced into progressive departments under various guises regardless of the views of unions and professional bodies. On scientific officers, the report fails to confirm reality and indeed almost resorts to wishful thinking. First class graduates are hard to come by and though they may not find difficulty in adjusting to medical work in teaching hospitals they do in adjusting to busy biochemistry departments in District General Hospitals. Can we really afford ample research facilities in order to attract staff?

In their evidence, pathologists suggested that their difficulties arose from inadequacies of the relevant H.M.C. in allocating sufficient funds. They felt that a committee of scientists at national and regional level should distribute resources but such committees could not increase the amount of money available. It is doubtful if they would distribute the money which is available any more efficiently than at present. Certainly their priorities would be different judging from the views of the College of Pathology who were reported as saying: 'The College is in a position to insist that the needs of trainees (pathologists) be considered before the short term needs of the laboratories . . .' (Editorial, 1966). Planning and co-ordination at regional level require knowledge and skill which are very scarce and which cannot be supplied in a brief management course at the King's Fund.

Biochemists implied in their evidence that many of their difficulties would disappear if they controlled their own laboratories both at hospital and regional level presumably free from the restraint of pathologists and the H.M.C. The report recommends that promotion to consultant status be open to biochemists, whether medically or non-medically qualified. The report seeks to 'wish away' the existing power structure in pathology departments with respect to pathologists and biochemists. Experience shows that clinicians, in general, resist any encroachment on their power status and there is no reason to believe pathologists are any different. Outside teaching hospitals a biochemistry department spends 95 per cent of its time and energy on routine work providing scientific information for clinicians. A Ph.D. is not much help in a job that is primarily concerned with organizing work and supervising staff. Some universities have employed graduates as laboratory supervisors with disappointing results.

Technicians are strongly in favour of Civil Service gradings but what they really mean is Civil Service salaries. This presents difficult problems, for the Ministry of Health have made it abundantly clear that any improvement will have to be made out of the existing income. Where will the money for higher salaries come from? One solution would be to employ fewer qualified technicians, for they tend to be employed on technical work requiring knowledge below the level of their qualifications. To reduce the number of technicians qualifying each year would further jeopardize the Institute of Medical Laboratory Technology who are already concerned about their future.

Before setting out to attract first class graduates, it would be worthwhile considering the recent work of Dr. Paul at an I.C.I.

146

research establishment. Using Herzberg's theory of motivation, he was able to induce the non-graduate technical staff, to be virtually as scientifically creative as science graduates in the same establishment. He is convinced that people at all levels have an enormous contribution to make and desperately want to make it, provided the organization gives them the framework within which to do so.

The Zuckerman Committee feel, as do the majority of scientists in the N.H.S., that more resources should be spent on hospital scientific services in spite of the fact that there are few complaints from hospital clinicians that their work is being hampered by the lack of scientific services. They noted the rapid increase in pathological requests but did not offer evidence of unsatisfied demand. It would be equally true to say that capacity or investment in pathology departments is increasing by 10 per cent per annum compared with hospital income which is increasing by 1 per cent per annum.

The report states that the committee set out to take stock of the present position but omitted to say that this was the present position as seen by a group of distinguished medically qualified scientists, physicians, biochemists and administrators. However, there are other ways of looking at organizations. Such diverse bodies as the Bank of England and the B.B.C. have called in management consultants to provide a fresh point of view. Others have asked social scientists to examine their organization—with great success. The total cost of the scientific services in the N.H.S., over 25 million pounds per annum, is large enough to benefit from the investigations of a top class management consultant team.

The report is deliberately vague, and rightly so, about job content and details of departmental organization at hospital level, as imposed solutions rarely work. All grades of staff should be involved in finding effective improvements in which they believe. It is important in this context to be aware of the difference between the public pronouncements of professional bodies and trade unions and what individual members feel in their own hospitals. Some professional bodies and unions are occasionally guilty of posturing either defensively or aggressively to impress their members.

The report represents the first step in what could be considered a scientific productivity agreement, as it calls for more efficiency, improved organization, greater flexibility and implies higher salaries. It goes on to say that 'we would expect the Minister, in consultation with staff interests and with the proposed new Scientific Council, would set up working parties to advise on the planning of particular services and on the integration of the present classes of staff into a new structure'.

Judging from the experience in industry, discussion on productivity agreements will show up any flaws in the management performance and structure, such as the gap between the management side of the Whitley Council, who negotiate agreements, and the H.M.C. which operates these agreements in each area. This gap has led to an 'indulgent pattern' of management such as overgrading and allowing 'on-call' fees to boost salaries. In a similar way pathologists are allowed domiciliary visits and fees from autopsies to boost their salaries. Discussions on productivity agreements will demonstrate any flaws in the skills of trade unions as negotiators and any gaps between their executive bodies and their members. It is also likely to create competition between professional bodies and trade unions and between trade unions themselves to show who is really representing scientists and technicians in such negotiations. These discussions will also demonstrate that management can no longer continue with a negative attitude, as in the past, only responding to pressure from trade unions or professional bodies. Finally, it is widely agreed that productivity agreements are not a 'once for all' process but a first step in a continuous process of improving the work climate.

The committee has made the common mistake of recommending only organizational and grading changes and ignoring the majority of problems which arise from the difficulties experienced by people as individuals and professionals in their jobs. This weakness is common to several reports on reorganization within the N.H.S. and is probably why such reports tend to get filed rather than implemented. The mistaken assumption is that the majority of present problems in the scientific services are due to faulty organization. This is not true, for the Central and Regional Pathology Advisory Committees could have undertaken most of the work of chief scientific officers if they had wished to do so. Much of the evidence submitted was concerned with faults in the organization but it is an accepted maxim in industrial psychology that complaints are often not related to the real problem.

Problems experienced by people as individuals in their jobs arise from changes in departmental organization, power and status, most of which originate from causes outside the scientific departments (Burns and Stalker, 1961). Changes in clinical practice have led to a substantial increase in the work-load of pathology departments and under pressure of work many pathologists have stopped signing pathology reports. Current clinical practice has created more technical work and rather less consultative work in pathology departments, so pathologists are developing into scientists rather than consultant clinical pathologists. Both of these factors together have altered the balance between pathologist and technician and imply a decrease in the status of pathologist and an increase in the status of those technicians who now sign reports and supervise the bulk of the technical work. Technology is so complex that today many pathologists can no longer supervise it and feel they are losing control to technicians and biochemists. Hospitals are complex organizations and short of money; this tends to increase the influence of the administrative chief technician. Pathologists, technicians and biochemists are barely aware of their new roles of supervisor, manager and technologist. All these changes taking place inside pathology and other departments can be seen to be the results of external change.

Revans (1964) stated that: 'Hospitals need to start learning to understand themselves better and this learning process can only take place when it is tackled voluntarily by those on the spot'. The same is true of scientific departments in hospitals. Staff of all grades will only make real and lasting improvements when they understand the problems and see what causes lie outside their department. It is disappointing that the report makes no mention of this and leaves staff to find out these things for themselves.

The report recommends that radiologists should continue to form part of the hospital clinical services but that radiographers should be assimilated into the new staffing structure and that career planning (presumably of radiographers) in consultation with the heads of departments should be the responsibility of the scientific services (presumably with the pathologist as chairman). This recommendation ignores the traditional power structure in hospitals. It may have been influenced by the relative position of pathology and radiology in medical schools and the relative power and influence of the College of Pathology and the Faculty of Radiology. It is difficult to think of an example in the N.H.S. where a scheme has been successfully implemented which cuts across the traditional structure. The sociological disturbances resulting may well involve costs which will considerably outweigh any benefits which may accrue from the recommendation.

There is little doubt that the present fragmented scientific services require reorganizing. However, in order to increase the chance of success and to minimize psychological and sociological disturbances, the reorganization should reinforce existing lines of development which are the realistic outcome of the 'political or power structure' in hospitals. A major effort has to be made, while implementing any new scheme, to recognize staff's needs as individuals and as professionals.

THE FUTURE SCIENTIFIC SERVICE

The future scientific service should be specifically designed to provide information and advice for all clinicians, not just those in hospitals, about their patients. This information can be divided into two broad groups one concerning cellular activity and the other the structure and function of the human body as a whole. The cellular function or micro system can be described in chemical terms, in architectural terms in the microscopic sense, or in functional terms. The techniques used to provide this information can originate in a number of scientific disciplines such as chemistry, physics, mathematics and physiology. The structure and function of the human body or macro system can be described in terms of physical structure, physical characteristics of components and mechanical ability to do work and to deal with air and water: that is, by lung and bladder functions. To provide this information until recently radiographic techniques and measurement of electrical current produced by muscle activity have been employed. More recently a number of new techniques have been introduced including ultrasonics, lasers and radioactive isotopes. These techniques are derived from one scientific discipline namely physics, though two major groups can be identified, one being instrument physics and the other radiation physics, such as radiography and radioactive isotopes. Each team could supervise or undertake the treatment of patients which involved complex or potentially dangerous equipment. The macro system team would include radiotherapy, as the basic science is identical. In larger hospitals each team would divide into specialized sub-teams to meet particular needs, as already happens in pathology departments.

This division of information required into groups leads to the postulation of two teams to provide it, one concerned with providing the information on the micro system and the other on the macro system of the human body. Each team would be organized on the lines suggested in previous chapters with a director, manager, technologist, technicians and laboratory assistants. The two teams would have to be co-ordinated on a regional basis to avoid duplication of effort or leaving some areas of technology or service untouched. There are currently two centrally organized services, the Public Health Laboratory Service and the Blood Transfusion Service which could be studied to discover how best to run the scientific service on a regional basis, thus enabling the more serious shortcomings of both to be avoided.

The organization for providing information on the micro system is well developed in the pathology departments particularly in view of the recent changes in the training system of technicians. The new H.N.C. emphasizes the cellular approach as the core of the syllabus is applied cellular biology The specialized subjects such as Haematology and Biochemistry are developed from this central theme. Within pathology departments the team has developed over the years to meet the range of skill and knowledge required with pathologist graduates and technicians with laboratory assistants not far away. Recruitment is flexible, staff can be recruited at various levels and yet promotion prospects are good for intelligent students as they can proceed through H.N.C. to a higher qualification and compete with graduates for technologists' posts. The new syllabus will enable qualified staff to be re-deployed and if necessary taught a new range of skills as the requirements of clinicians alter and new techniques are introduced. It would, for example, be relatively simple to train the specialist technician required in bio-engineering in this manner.

The organization for providing information on the macro system is less well developed and is still to a large extent centred on technology and becoming increasingly fragmented. The largest department is Radiography, still using one principal technique; with a number of very much smaller units such as Electrocardiography, Electro-encephalography, Audiology, Physiological Measurement and Physiotherapy departments undertaking Myography. In the teaching hospitals and a small number of general hospitals medical physics departments are well established. Recently new departments have been set up, using radioactive isotopes in various techniques, with a confusing range of names—for example, department of nuclear medicine—which sometimes appear to be competing with each other. Radiography departments have failed to acquire a group of graduate technologists and only have consultant radiologists with medical qualifications and technicians with a qualification approximately equal to O.N.C. The teams in Medical Physics, Radiotherapy and Nuclear Medicine Departments vary as some are directed by graduates and others by medically qualified staff with technicians who are either radiographers or physics technicians. Until recently the physics technicians had no specified qualifications and a very varied training. The ambitions of the professional groups are preventing the various departments from coalescing into more effective units. Recruitment for technicians is only at student level and career prospects are limited by the small size of departments. The radiographer's training with its emphasis on techniques, makes it difficult to re-deploy them and although physics technicians are developing a common training course it will not produce qualified staff until 1972. Recruiting will always be a problem in the smaller groups such as E.G.G. and E.E.G. technicians because of low level of qualifications and poor career prospects. This situation is slowing down the development of medical physics and bio-engineering.

This organization of two teams would have the advantage of being evolutionary in that pathology and radiology departments could be developed to form them instead of attempting to create a new organization as has been suggested. Analysis of the development of the N.H.S. and pathology departments indicates that the most successful methods of introducing new ideas have been evolutionary rather than revolutionary.

If professional groups are prepared to consider the scientific service as a real service for clinicians as well as offering status and career prospects for themselves, they could make an important contribution to its development. They need to understand and appreciate the concept of service to clinicians, to understand the hospital as a bureaucratic system with its advantages and disadvantages and come to realize that organizational effectiveness and efficiency are not incompatible with a satisfying professional job. In a similar way the hospital planners and administrators should be prepared to consider not only how a scientific service should be organized in terms of efficiency but also how it can provide an environment in which pathologists, graduates and technicians can find real job satisfaction and satisfy their needs as individuals. The planners and managers could look at the skills and ambitions of the three groups and distinguish between managing professionals and providing an environment and resources for them. Pathology departments as organizations should take account of what the clinicians want—an effective performance; what the H.M.C. wants —an efficient service; and what the staff want—a sense of belonging and of doing a worthwhile job which means professional freedom and status. Above all, pathology departments should, if they are to be effective, attempt to match the needs of providing an effective and efficient service with the human needs of the staff giving the service.

REFERENCES

A.C.P. Broadsheet No. 30 (1964). London; College of Pathologists.

Association of Scientific, Technical and Managerial Staff (1968). *Br. Hosp. Jnl. soc. Serv. Rev.,* 1087.

Bagrit, L. (1966). *The Age of Automation.* Harmondsworth; Penguin.

Battersby, A. (1967). *Network Analysis for Planning and Scheduling,* 2nd Ed. London; Macmillan.

Bennett, C. H. N. (1967). *Br. Hosp. Jnl. soc. Serv. Rev.,* pp. 19 and 1163.

Bold, A. M. and Corrin, B. (1965). *Br. med. J.,* 2, 1051.

British Standards Institute: Glossary of Terms in Work Study, No. 3138, Amended (Pl) 4585 (1962). London.

Brown, J. A. C. (1954). *The Social Psychology of Industry.* Harmondsworth; Penguin.

Brown, W. (1960). *Exploration in Management.* London; Heinemann.

Burns, T. and Stalker, G. M. (1961). *Management of Innovation.* London; Tavistock.

Cappell, D. F. (1960). *Lancet,* 2, 864.

Carter, M. P. (1966). *Into Work,* London; Penguin.

Cook, R. V. (1967). *Br. med. J.,* 2, 129.

Crichton, A. (1963). *Disappointed Expectations.* Welsh Hospital Board.

Darmady, E. M. (1964). *J. clin. Path.,* 17, 477.

Davey, E. M. (1954). *Lancet,* 2, 1223.

Department of Scientific and Industrial Research (1964). *Ergonomics in Industry.* London; D.S.I.R.

Dible, J. H. (1957). *J. Path. Bact.,* 73, 1.

Dyke, S. C. (1940). *Lancet,* 1, 86.

— (Ed.) (1964). *Recent Advances in Clinical Pathology,* Vol. 4. London; Churchill.

Editorial (1966). *Lancet,* 2, 93.

Enquiry into the Flow of Candidates in Science and Technology into Higher Education. Cmnd, 3541. (1968). London; H.M.S.O.

Foster, W. D. (1961). *A Short History of Clinical Pathology.* Edinburgh and London; Livingstone.

Fraser, J. Munro (1965). *Industrial Psychology.* London; Pergamon.

Gould, J. C. (1966). *J. clin. Path.,* 19, 408.

Herzberg, F., Mausner, B. and Snyderman, B. (1959). *The Motivation to Work.* New York; John Wiley.

Human Problems of Innovation. Problems of Progress in Industry, No. 5 (1967). London; H.M.S.O.

Imperial Chemical Industries (1962). Monograph No. 1. 'Mathematical Trend Curve: An Aid to Forecasting.' Edinburgh; Oliver and Boyd.

— (1964). Monograph No. 2. 'Short-term Forecasting.' Edinburgh; Oliver and Boyd.

Leading Article (1957). *Br. med. J.,* 2, 1419.

— (1967). *J. clin. Path.,* 20, 1.

Lockyer, K. G. (1964). *An Introduction to Critical Path Analysis.* London; Pitman.
Lupton, T. (1966). *Management and the Social Sciences.* London; Hutchinson.
Maier, N. (1961). *Frustration.* Michigan; Cresset.
McGregor, D. (1960). *The Human Side of Enterprise.* New York; McGraw-Hill.
Ministry of Health (1965). *Hospital Building Notes for Pathology Departments,* London; H.M.S.O.
— (1967). *The Hospital Services Organization and Management Report,* No. 10. London; H.M.S.O.
— (1968a). *Hospital Scientific and Technical Services.* London; H.M.S.O.
— (1968b). *Circular. Management in the Eighties.* 28(68). London; H.M.S.O.
Mitchell, W. A. (1933). Survey of Pathology and Bacteriology Laboratory Assistants Association. Unpublished.
Optimum Purchasing Policy, Paper No. 4 (1962). Oxford Regional Hospital Board. Operational Research Unit.
Redfurn, P. (1967). C.A.S. Occasional Paper No. 5. 'The Input-output Analysis and its Application to Education and Manpower Planning.' London; H.M.S.O.
Reid Report (1956).
Report, Annual (1958–1966). Of the Chief Medical Officer of the Ministry of Health. London; H.M.S.O.
— Crowther (1959, 1960). London; H.M.S.O.
— of a Scottish Hospital Service Committee (1966a). *Administrative Practice of Hospital Boards in Scotland,* London; H.M.S.O.
— of a Committee, Department of Health and Social Security (1966b). *Hospital Supplies Organisations.* London; H.M.S.O.
— (1966c). *Senior Nursing Staff Structure.* London; H.M.S.O.
— of a Standing Advisory Committee (1966d). *Training of Pathologists and Recognition of Laboratories.* London; College of Pathologists.
— of a Joint Working Party (1967). *The Organisation of Medical Work in Hospitals.* London; H.M.S.O.
— on Data Processing in Clinical Pathology (1968). *J. clin. Path.,* **21**, 231.
Report of I.M.L.T. (1947). *Bull. Inst. med. Lab. Technol.,* **13**, 6.
— Annual, of I.M.L.T. (1958). *Gaz. Inst. med. Lab. Technol.,* **14**.
— of I.M.L.T. (1963). *Gaz. Inst. med. Lab. Technol.,* **7**, 138.
— of I.M.L.T. (1965). *Gaz. Inst. med. Lab. Technol.,* **9**, 1.
Revans, R. W. (1964). *Br. med. J.,* **2**, 1456.
— (1965). *Science and the Manager.* London; Macdonald.
Schein, E. H. (1965). *Organizational Psychology.* London; Prentice-Hall.
Sprott, W. J. H. (1958). *Human Groups.* Harmondsworth; Penguin.

REFERENCES

Stevens, R. (1966). *Medical Practice in Modern England*. Newhaven, Conn; Yale University Press.

Supervisory Training: A New Approach for Management (1966). London; H.M.S.O.

Survey (1965). Association of Scientific Workers.

Walsh, D. B. (1967). *Br. med. J.*, **2**, 447.

Weaver, J. and Puente, J. (1964). *Acta Cytol.*, **8**, 270.

Whitehead, T. (1967). *Proc. Ass. clin. Biochemists*, **1**, 122.

Zuckerman, Sir S. (1968). *Hospital Scientific and Technical Services*. London; H.M.S.O.

INDEX